Calm &
SENSE

WENDY LEEDS

Calm &
SENSE

A Woman's Guide to
Living Anxiety-Free

Calm & Sense: A Woman's Guide to Living Anxiety-Free
© 2020 Wendy Leeds

Published by Calm Day Publishing

Second edition print ISBN: 978-0-9999015-2-6
Second edition ebook ISBN: 978-0-9999015-3-3

Illustrations by Meg Joyce
Cover design by Liz Schreiter
Interior design by Andrea Reider
Editing and book production by Reading List Editorial:
readinglisteditorial.com

AUTHOR'S NOTE

ALL THE case studies in this book have been created to high-light the tools and techniques listed in this book and are based on fictional characters and circumstances. Any resemblance to people living or dead is purely coincidental.

The information in this book is not designed to replace medical or psychiatric treatment or as a substitute for medical advice. If you are in need of medical health services, please seek professional advice. Use of this book does not establish a therapist/practitioner-patient relationship.

If you're suffering from severe trauma, anxiety co-occuring with depression, an eating disorder, or any disorder that is making your life beyond miserable, please reach out to your health care provider for help.

Suicidal Thoughts or Plans

If you're thinking about killing yourself, or if you have a plan to kill or harm yourself or anyone else, please put down this book and go call for help. NOW!

- Call a trusted friend.
- Call 911.
- Go to the nearest emergency room.
- Call this suicide prevention number 1-800-273-TALK (8255).
- Visit http://www.suicidepreventionlifeline.org.

This book is dedicated to my husband, Thomas F. Leeds.
Thank you for making this dream possible.

Contents

Part Three: Reframe Your Anxiety

Part Four: Tame Your Anxiety

Introduction

I knew that if I allowed fear to overtake me, my journey was doomed. Fear, to a great extent, is born of a story we tell ourselves, and so I chose to tell myself a different story from the one women are told. I decided I was safe. I was strong. I was brave. Nothing could vanquish me.

—Cheryl Strayed, best-selling author of
Wild, Tiny Beautiful Things, and *Brave Enough*

JUST AFTER two o'clock on a beautiful Friday afternoon late in June, I got the call from my doctor that every woman dreads. I had breast cancer.

I remember holding the phone to my ear long after the call was over, frozen with fear. When I was finally able to move again, I couldn't stop shaking. I still remember the shock at hearing the words and the cold, hard terror at what lay ahead.

Within a week of diagnosis, I underwent surgery. Two weeks later, I started six months of chemotherapy, which was eventually followed by four more surgeries.

Physically, the treatment for breast cancer was difficult, but I knew there was an end in sight to *that* pain. Emotionally, the fear and worry went on for years.

What if the cancer came back? What if it spread? What would happen to my children? My family? How would I be able to deal with it a second time? Every new ache or pain terrified me.

Now, I was no stranger to anxiety. I'd grown up in an anxious family, and I'd worried my way through life. But this was different. This fear was a weight in my gut that kept me awake nights and haunted my days.

For years I continued to walk through my life on autopilot, thinking there was something wrong with me for not being able to deal with this black fear, believing it was something to be ashamed of, a dark, terrible secret I couldn't share with anyone.

And then someone suggested I try reading a book by Cheryl Richardson. Someone else suggested I read something by Louise Hay. And I found Norman Vincent Peale, Susan Jeffers, Tony Robbins, Joan Borysenko, Albert Ellis, John Bradshaw, Martha Beck, Aaron Beck, David Burns, and many others.

Once I started reading, I couldn't stop. I read everything I could get my hands on about anxiety. I was comforted to find I wasn't alone with my fear and excited to learn there was something I could do about it.

Eventually, I tried almost all the techniques I was reading about. And I began replacing my worry and fear with a sense of peace that came from the inside out.

A few years later, I went back to graduate school to study psychology. At graduation, I joined a small psychotherapy practice and was able to use the tools I'd learned over the years to help my clients heal their anxiety. I was on top of the world. I remember the joy of thinking that I'd finally created the life I'd always longed for. But the story doesn't end there.

On a Monday night in June, at 7:30 p.m. to be precise, my doctor called to tell me I had leukemia.

Really? Cancer again?

All I could think of was the suffering I'd gone through after the last diagnosis. The pain and exhaustion of chemo and surgery and the fear . . .

I wondered how I was ever going to get through all that again. It wasn't the physical trauma of treatment that scared me. It was *that fear.*

And then I realized it could be different this time. I now had an entire tool kit filled with new ways of thinking, lifestyle changes I could make, and physical techniques I could use to make myself feel better. I just had to start using them.

I didn't have to suffer this time. What a relief. What a difference.

This time I asked for and got lots of help. I found an amazing health and wellness coach, who taught me to eat well and to take care of myself with a loving heart.

I went to therapy. I went to an acupuncturist. I called on friends for support. I practiced gratitude, journaling, emotional freedom technique (EFT), cognitive behavioral therapy (CBT), affirmations, yoga, breathing, and most of the other things you're going to read about in this book.

And while I suffered physically, this time I didn't feel alone or afraid. This time I had the tools and techniques to handle anything that happened to me!

This Is for All of Us

I'm excited to be able to share what I've learned over all these years with you and every other anxious woman on the planet. And there are a lot of us.

Women in this country are twice as likely to be diagnosed with anxiety, and we're much more likely to be put on medication than our male counterparts. One out of four American women is prescribed medication for a mental health condition, as opposed to 15 percent of men.

Far too many of us have been suffering in silence.

But not anymore!

Today we're going to start talking about our anxiety and working together to heal the fears that keep us up at night and limit our lives.

No more hiding. No more shame. No more pretending everything's all right when it isn't.

Together we're going to explore *your* anxiety. We're going to name it, look at what causes it, and then together we're going to find the anxiety-easing tools that work best for you.

Calm and Sense is divided into the following parts:

1. **Name Your Anxiety** defines anxiety.
2. **Claim Your Anxiety** explores the specifics of your particular anxiety.
3. **Reframe Your Anxiety** discusses how to ease anxiety by changing your thoughts.
4. **Tame Your Anxiety** offers specific tools and techniques to physically manage your anxiety.
5. **Create Your Own Anxiety-Free Day,** an appendix, suggests ways for you to put the tools you've been reading about to work in your daily life.

How to Use This Book

You can read *Calm and Sense* cover to cover or jump right in and try some of these amazing techniques for yourself. If what you try doesn't work for you—no worries. Try something else. Do things twice. Do them your own way. Let go of judgment and allow yourself to enjoy you for a change.

You can't do this wrong.

And that includes the decision of whether or not to take medication for your anxiety. For many women, medication is the only answer to feeling better. It may be the right answer for you, too. I've seen firsthand how the right medication can save lives, offer hope, and restore quality of life in a way nothing else can. So if you and your health care professional decide that medication is what you need, take the medication.

But why not consider trying some of the techniques in this book along with the medication for an even better outcome? Be sure to let your doctor know what you're doing. The very best partnerships are the ones that allow open and honest communication, so don't hold back. Your doc is probably very smart, but she can't read your mind. Let her know how you feel and what you're doing to help yourself feel better.

Whatever you do, if a technique or tool doesn't feel right for you, don't use it. Healing anxiety should *always* make you feel better. Please, no more punishing yourself by setting impossible goals or berating yourself for not being braver or smarter, and no more self-abuse for the time wasted. I promise that you have what it takes to make healthy changes to your life.

Nobody can go back and start a new beginning,
but anyone can start today and make a new ending.

—Maria Robinson, early childhood expert
and author of *The Feeling Child*

PART ONE

NAME YOUR ANXIETY

If I asked you to name all the things that you love,
how long would it take to claim yourself?

—Author unknown

CHAPTER I

The Anxious Brain

*If depression is, as Winston Churchill famously described,
a "black dog that follows the sufferer around," anxiety is a
feral cat that springs from nowhere, sinks its claws into skin,
and hisses invectives until nothing else exists.*

—Kat Kinsman, food editor and author of *Hi, Anxiety*

ANXIETY BEGINS in the amygdala. I think of the amygdala as a kind of communication hub in your brain. It receives information from all your senses. In a split second, it decides what that information means to you and your survival; then it sends that information on to other parts of your brain.

As Regina Bailey explains in her article "Amygdala's Location and Function," the amygdala is "an almond-shaped mass of nuclei [mass of cells] located deep within the temporal lobe of the brain . . . [It's] involved in many of our emotions and motivations, particularly those that are related to survival. The amygdala is involved in the processing of emotions such as fear, anger, and pleasure."

meditation to calm her neocortex. Georgia found that using two approaches helped bring a new sense of calm into her life.

The amygdala's initial fear response seems to work the same in everyone's brains, but recent research suggests that long-term anxiety can show up differently in women's brains.

Now, it's important to remember we're talking in generalities here. Our brains all share some commonalities, but in the end they're all unique. And as with all gender differences, no one way of thinking is better or worse than the other. All differences have advantages and disadvantages.

Let's take a look at some of those differences.

Gender Differences in Our Brains

Rose and Dan had been married for sixteen years, but lately they'd just been "going through the motions."

When Dan brought up the subject of divorce, they agreed to see a therapist in a last-ditch effort to save their marriage. At their first session, the therapist asked them to share their complaints about each other, and they didn't hold back.

Rose complained, "Dan won't fight with me. When he gets angry, he just clams up, and that drives me crazy. How can we settle anything if we don't talk? We just don't communicate."

"I'd say she communicates enough for both of us," Dan shot back. "She never lets anything go. Every time we fight, she brings up things I did ten years ago. There's this list of 'bad things Dan has done' she runs through every time I do something that ticks her off."

The therapist nodded. "It sounds like you both react to conflict in different ways, and some of that may be due to the fact that, in general, men's and women's brains tend to react to stress differently."

"What do you mean?" Rose asked.

The therapist motioned to Dan. "For years we believed that the human reaction to stress was either 'fight or flight,'" the therapist explained. "But recent research proves that's the *male's* response to danger or conflict. In the male brain, the circuit of aggression is connected to areas in the brain linked to physical action. So males tend to respond by acting—either they stand and fight, or they run."

The therapist turned to Rose. "But in female brains, that circuit of aggression is more connected to areas of the brain for thinking, feeling, and talking. So the *female's* response to danger or conflict may be what we call 'tend and befriend.' After the amygdala's initial 'uh-oh' response to fear (which we all share), women tend to deal with danger, conflict, or anxiety by bonding, connecting, communicating, and reaching out."

The therapist continued. "So the female brain says, 'Go ahead, talk it out,' while the male brain says, 'Don't talk; do something,' or it disengages entirely."

Rose looked at Dan. "That sounds just like us."

Dan nodded in agreement. "When I'm stressed, all I want to do is avoid human contact. And I've never been able to figure out why she didn't want to avoid *me*." He smiled at Rose. "But if we're wired differently, that finally makes some sense."

As Rose returned his smile, the therapist continued. "And the differences in your brains don't stop there. It turns out, women and men remember things differently. Research shows that in women, there tends to be more blood flow in the part of the brain that processes emotions and relates them to events.

"This causes women to revisit and ruminate on emotional memories more than men. So women are more likely to remember and rethink the past in greater detail, going over things again and again, as if repeatedly watching a full-length movie."

Dan looked at Rose as if beginning to see her in a different light. "So that's why she keeps harping on something long after it makes any sense to bring it up." He looked back at the therapist. "And I bet the way she thinks about things over and over is making her really anxious, too."

What has Mark learned? That it's okay to feel fear and keep going. "You're capable of overcoming obstacles. Go ahead, you can do this." When he gets older, chances are he'll trust himself to take action. And action is one of the best ways to overcome anxiety.

They've learned to deal with their fear differently. Mark has learned to meet his problems head-on, while Mary has been taught to retreat, worry, and complain rather than take action and confront her fear.

Of course, these are all generalizations. Views on traditional gender roles are shifting, and things may have been very different for you.

Take a moment and think back to what *you* learned on the playground.

How What We Learned on the Playground Affects Our Anxiety

Now let's take a look at how all the lessons we learned when we were younger can translate into the anxiety we feel today. You may be surprised to learn how these early experiences impact what you think about yourself today, how you treat yourself, and how you see the world around you.

Work

Jen has grown up to both fear and avoid confrontation. When she was passed over for a richly deserved promotion at work, she didn't have the courage to speak up for herself. Instead, she lay awake nights, staring at the ceiling, telling herself she probably couldn't have done the job anyway.

Serena knew she deserved to be paid more and finally found the courage to bring up a raise during her quarterly review. But when her boss said no, Serena decided to "not rock the boat" and didn't ask again. Instead she continued to bite her nails and drink a second glass of wine at night to keep her feelings of failure and fear at bay.

Phyllis dreamed of starting her own business. When she shared those dreams with her girlfriends, they told her scary stories about failure. They reminded her she was lucky to have a job and it's better to be safe than sorry. Phyllis listened and never took a single step toward her dream.

Sound familiar?

Women worry much more about work than men. We have to work harder to get the credit we deserve, and some of us still have to deal with discrimination and harassment on the job.

Money

Nora got up every morning worrying about money. She went to bed every night still worrying about being to be able to pay all her bills, concerned about how to keep a roof over her head, afraid she'd never be able to retire. "I'm just not good with money," she told herself. "And I don't know what to do about it."

Nora is like a lot of us. Women are much more likely to lose sleep worrying over money, and it's no wonder.

We're also more likely to live in poverty than men. Women are still paid only three-quarters of what men are paid for the same job. We're the ones who take time off to care for children and aging parents. And, as a rule, we have less money set aside for retirement.

To add insult to injury, we're likely to live seven years longer than men, so we need to have *more* money than men to cover those extra years in retirement.

Of course we worry about outliving our money.

But it's not just the things outside us that make us worry about money. What we're taught about ourselves and our abilities to handle money can also be a factor in our lack of financial well-being.

When a major financial institution asked high school students how good they were with money and math, the boys generally answered, "We're pretty good." The girls answered, "We're not very good." But here's the kicker. Both groups knew the same information. The girls just weren't as confident in themselves or their abilities.

Relationships

Carol was exhausted. She was caring for her two teenage sons and her aging mother while holding down a full-time job. She felt responsible for everyone else's health and happiness but her own, and it took a serious health scare to remind her that she needed to take care of herself.

And Carol's not alone. Studies show that it's much more important for women to have good relationships with friends and family than men. When our relationships are on the rocks, we worry and work feverishly to restore them.

We're the ones who are more likely to worry about the health of our partners and our children. We run ourselves ragged trying to balance our roles as mother, daughter, partner, friend, and professional, attempting to do it all, have it all, and make sure everyone else is healthy and happy.

Time

Kim got up every morning, made herself a cup of coffee, and started folding laundry.

By the time her partner and two children came down for breakfast, she'd planned dinner, packed lunches, answered work emails, emptied the dishwasher, and poured the cereal.

As she headed out the door for work, Kim was already running behind and felt like the day was "getting away from her." No matter how hard and fast she worked, Kim knew she was never going to get everything done. The laundry would multiply overnight. The dirty dishes would magically appear in the sink, and the school always scheduled their concerts on nights she had to work late.

Kim told her best friend, "I'd be the queen of anxiety if I had any time left over in my day to worry."

If you feel the same way, join the club.

According to a survey done by the Pew Research Center, women do more than their share of the housework and childcare, even if we work full time. And according to a study conducted by *Real Simple* and the Families and Work Institute, 52 percent of American women have less than ninety minutes a day of free time, and 29 percent of us have less than forty-five minutes a day to relax. And 46 percent of us say that what free time we do have is interrupted.

Sound familiar?

We don't get enough sleep. We don't take the time to eat a healthy diet. We don't have time to hit the gym. We give up doing the things that fill our souls with peace and we suffer for it.

We're told we can have it all, and we're encouraged to do it all. We're told we can be great mothers and successful businesswomen, we can look great and feel great, and we can still have time left over to have fun. And when we don't, or can't, we worry we're not good enough.

What About You?

Maybe you've recognized yourself in the stories above, or maybe your anxiety comes from some other cause. If you're not sure where your anxiety comes from, don't worry. We're going to spend some time together getting to really know your anxiety in detail. Then we're going to get down to the business of helping you deal with that anxiety in ways that will finally set you free from that fear.

But first let's look at some of the effects anxiety can have on you and your life.

CHAPTER 3

How Women Worry: Signs, Symptoms, and Effects of Anxiety

My struggle with anxiety has almost always been tied to my femaleness. It's closely linked to negative feelings about my body and physical attractiveness, dating, and the irrational fear that I'm going to end up childless and alone.

—Emma Gray, editor at HuffPost and author of
A Girl's Guide to Joining the Resistance

S O HOW does anxiety show up in our lives? How and when did it start? How long will it last? That answer is different for everyone. But let's take a look at how anxiety showed up for two very different women and how they've learned to deal with it.

Danica (Generalized Anxiety Disorder)

Danica was a worrier. As a child, she lived in a constant state of dread that something awful was about to happen. She worried about doing well in school. She worried whether or not her friends liked her. She was afraid of the dark and terrified she or her parents would get sick and die.

She dragged herself to school every Monday morning and lived all day in fear that her teacher would call on her. She worried that no one would sit with her at lunch and that she'd miss the afternoon bus home. The night before a test, Danica would lie awake, going over the material in her head until she knew it by heart. But the next day, when she started reading the test questions, her mind would go blank and she would tense up until her teeth hurt.

Danica graduated from high school near the top of her class and dreamed of opening her own restaurant. But she settled on attending the local junior college near her home rather than risk leaving her small town to attend the culinary school of her dreams.

People often described Danica as shy, funny, and creative, but she didn't feel like that. She felt like an imposter and thought she was the only one who worried all the time. She didn't have any hope of changing her worried ways until she took a psychology course during her sophomore year in college.

When she started reading about GAD, Danica felt as if the words were describing *her*, as if the author could see inside her and knew exactly how she felt and what she was thinking.

She was both surprised and excited to read she wasn't the only one spending her life dreading school, fearing the dark, avoiding social situations, and being terrified of getting sick. And she was delighted to learn that although GAD was chronic, it was treatable. Lots of women were living with GAD and doing well. And for the first time, she began to wonder what her life would look like without the constant weight of worry.

Danica went to her college counselor, and together they created a plan to help Danica deal with her GAD. With her counselor's encouragement, Danica read everything she could get her hands on about GAD and found effective ways to ease her fears, including taking a beginner's yoga class and blogging about her experience online with other women with GAD.

She learned to use her sense of humor to challenge her negative thinking and to replace her negative thoughts of the future with more positive, upbeat possibilities.

As she learned new ways of dealing with her GAD, Danica began to consider the possibility of going to culinary school after all.

Liz (Panic Attacks)

At forty-seven, Liz had never been nervous a day in her life, until late one Thursday afternoon. As she pulled up in front of the grocery store, Liz's heart suddenly started to race. Her chest tightened until she felt like she was suffocating to death. Terrified she was having a heart attack, Liz drove herself to the local emergency room. After a series of tests, the doctors told her they couldn't find anything wrong with her physically. They suggested she was having a panic attack and urged her to check in with her primary care physician (PCP).

Liz hesitated, not wanting to "make a fuss over nothing." But when the attacks continued, she started having trouble leaving home. She canceled social plans and made excuses to avoid going out. When Liz realized her fear of having a panic attack was taking over her life, she finally made and kept an appointment with her doctor.

She was relieved when her PCP reassured her that she wasn't "losing her mind" or "making it all up." The panic attacks she was experiencing were probably caused by the fluctuations in her hormones as she headed into perimenopause.

The good news was that these panic attacks would lessen as her hormones evened out. The bad news was that Liz needed to come up with a plan to deal with both the attacks and, even more debilitating, her fear of having an attack. Her doctor suggested that Liz start by keeping a daily log to help her identify the triggers for her panic. After just a few days, Liz noticed she was much more anxious after her morning cup of coffee, and two days later she had a full-blown panic attack at the end of a long, tiring day.

Knowing that both caffeine and being overly tired were triggers for panic helped Liz make lifestyle changes that cut down on the number of panic attacks she experienced.

She also learned a number of techniques to help her deal with the attacks after they'd started. She used acupressure points and repeated focus phrases like "I'm all right," "I know what this is; I know this will pass quickly," "I'm already feeling better," and "I will be fine" until she felt calmer.

Once Liz had a plan for heading off attacks and for meeting an attack head-on, she was able to move past her fears and get back to living her best life.

Symptoms of Anxiety

Anxiety can start at any time during our lives. It can come on gradually or all of a sudden. It can be long-term or a passing thing. The symptoms can be so mild you hardly notice them, or so severe they make your life miserable. You may experience a range of symptoms, and those symptoms may change over time.

Let's take a look at some common symptoms of anxiety.

Physical Symptoms:

- Sweating
- Nausea
- Trembling
- Tingling
- Twitching
- Pulsing

- Burning
- Tension anywhere in your body
- Headaches
- Dizziness
- Weakness
- A pounding heart
- Chest pain
- Shortness of breath/smothering

Emotional Symptoms:

- Feeling restless
- Feeling tense and jumpy
- Feeling irritable
- Feeling exhausted
- Feeling like you're all alone

Cognitive Symptoms:

When you're anxious, you may have trouble thinking at all. You may have racing thoughts. You may also have thoughts like the following:

- I'm going crazy.
- I might lose control or become incapacitated.
- I have to worry because if I worry hard enough and long enough, I'll be safe.
- I won't be able to handle what is ahead for me.
- Something awful is going to happen.
- I'm going to end up old and alone and broke.
- I'm going to die.
- We're all going to die.
- ARGH!!!!!

How many of these symptoms do you experience in your daily life? Have you ever stopped to consider the impact these symptoms have on your life? Have you considered how your fears limit the way you experience the world around you?

Let's take a look at what these symptoms are costing you, then put together a plan to do something about it!

CHAPTER 4

The Price We Pay
for Being Anxious

*Women are nearly twice as likely as men to
develop anxiety, because they have twice
as much to be anxious about.*

—Susan Rinkunas, senior editor at *VICE*

ANXIETY CAN have a tremendous impact on our lives. It can cause difficulties in relationships and can create struggles at work, at school, and at home. Anxiety can make you miss important moments in your life, and it can make you feel lonely, lost, and hopeless.

How about you? Have you ever stopped to consider the price you pay for your anxiety?

Here are the stories of two women who realized how much their anxiety was costing them and did something about it.

Whitney

Whitney was terrified of driving over the long, high drawbridge that spanned the river dividing her hometown. Just the thought of driving up and over the arching four-lane highway made her hands sweat and her whole body shake. If she needed to get to the other side of town, Whitney would drive nearly forty-five minutes out of her way to avoid the ten-minute trip over the bridge. That meant she didn't often see her friends who lived on the other side of town. She rarely shopped over there, and she put off going to the dentist and doctor because it took her so long to get to their offices.

Whitney had lots of excuses for not crossing that bridge. She told anyone who'd listen that she had so many friends, she didn't have time to see everyone. She had more choices when she shopped online. She didn't need to see her health care professionals, because she was "as healthy as a horse," and besides, she liked taking the "scenic route."

When Whitney was offered her dream job on the other side of town, she turned it down. She knew she couldn't make the long drive twice a day. But she told everyone that the job was too demanding, and she didn't want to work "those kinds of hours."

In spite of all her excuses, Whitney knew her fear of driving across the bridge was literally keeping her prisoner on her side of the river. And she continued to pretend everything was okay until her son and his newly pregnant wife moved to the other side of the river.

Then Whitney couldn't pretend anymore. If she wanted to continue seeing her son and his young family several times a week, Whitney knew she was going to have to find a way to be able to drive across the bridge.

The day after she heard about her expected grandchild, Whitney went online and started reading. Right away, she learned that she wasn't the only one afraid of bridges. There were lots of people who had a similar fear, and in fact, that fear had a name: gephyrophobia.

She also learned that her fellow gephyrophobes had come up with some sensible solutions to deal with that fear. Drawing from their suggestions, Whitney put together a tool kit of breathing techniques, acupressure points, and affirmations she could use when she felt even the tiniest bit of panic at the idea of crossing the bridge. She practiced the techniques as often as possible. She knew it usually took six to nine months to successfully get over gephyrophobia, and she was determined to be able to cross the bridge in time to welcome that first grandchild.

Next Whitney began to visualize successfully driving across the bridge.

When she finally felt comfortable with her visualizations, Whitney decided she was ready to ride across the bridge with another driver. She asked her sister to drive her, then created a playlist of great music she could listen to as they crossed the bridge. Early one Tuesday morning, Whitney put in her earbuds and focused on the music as she and her sister made their first successful drive across the bridge.

For the next few months, Whitney continued to ride back and forth over the bridge with her sister or a friend, each time focusing on her music, affirmations, and breathing techniques to keep herself calm.

When it came time for her first drive across the bridge, Whitney asked her sister to ride with her. She turned up her music full blast and sang along with that music at the top of her lungs, all the way across the bridge.

Later, her sister told her about the strange looks they'd gotten from some of other drivers as Whitney sang her way across the bridge. "They were looking at you like you're crazy," her sister said. "But the truth is, you did a great job. And I'm really proud of you."

Six weeks later, Whitney drove all the way across the bridge on her own to welcome her new granddaughter.

Lena

For Lena, feelings of suddenly being overwhelmed by life seemed to show up out of nowhere. At thirty-six, she was being treated for infertility, and not being able to get pregnant was all she could think about. She felt guilty for putting off having a family until she'd established herself in her career as an architect.

She felt guilty for not being able to give her husband, Jeff, a child, and she was sick of seeing smiling pregnant women everywhere she went. Not to mention all the medical tests, interventions, and uncertainty that lay ahead.

As the time neared for her first treatment, Lena's appetite seemed to vanish, until all she was eating was yogurt and orange juice. She lost weight. She and Jeff argued so much, she began to wonder if their ten-year marriage would survive the IVF treatment.

And then the migraines started.

Lena had always been proud of her ability to soldier on no matter how tough things got. She wasn't one of those women who went running for help at the first sign of trouble. But the headaches were so ferocious, she started missing work and she felt like crying all the time.

So at her next appointment, Lena reluctantly mentioned the migraines to the doctor. To her surprise, the doctor told her her headaches could be a symptom of anxiety, as well as conditions like heart disease, chronic respiratory diseases like asthma and COPD, and gastrointestinal conditions like IBS. She also mentioned that anxiety leads to eating disorders, insomnia, and addictions to things like drugs, alcohol, nicotine, gambling, video games, or shopping.

When the doctor went on to question Lena about her loss of appetite, Lena finally broke down and admitted she was a wreck both physically and emotionally. She told the doctor about the troubles in her relationship with her husband, her inability to think about anything but her infertility, and her guilt.

The doctor nodded and explained that anxiety can not only cause physical disorders, but it can also play havoc in relationships and create real problems at work.

Relieved to hear she wasn't sick or crazy, Lena was open to the doctor's suggestions for ways to start feeling better. Together they came up with a plan that included couples counseling to help heal Lena's relationship with Jeff, a meditation group to help Lena find peace and stay in the moment, and a consultation with a nutritionist to help Lena get back on track with her eating plan.

In time Lena added a weekly massage to help ease her physical stress. And she and Jeff scheduled a romantic getaway to Cape Cod.

The counseling helped bring Lena and Jeff closer than ever. The meditation and healthy eating plan helped Lena feel better physically, and within a few weeks her migraines vanished.

Six months later, Lena got good news. She was pregnant. Although the doctor said no one's sure exactly what role anxiety plays in fertility, Lena believed that the steps she took to ease her anxiety and feel better physically helped in the process.

You

Like Whitney, have you missed any events or important appointments? Your prom? A special reunion? Your best friend's wedding? Medical appointments? That movie everyone's talking about?

Has your performance suffered at work or at school? Maybe, like Whitney, you passed up a job you really wanted, or maybe anxiety is keeping you from leaving a job you hate. Did you struggle in school because of anxiety? Did you give up on yourself at some point?

Or maybe, like Lena, you're suffering physical symptoms. Are you having trouble sleeping or are you eating too much or too little? Are you smoking? Drinking or shopping too much? Maybe you're running too much, working too much, or sleeping all the time.

How about your relationships? Are you afraid to speak up for what you want in a relationship? Are you staying in a relationship that no longer works because you're afraid of being alone? Is anxiety keeping you from meeting new people, maybe even someone special? Does being anxious keep you from getting close to the people around you?

Take a minute and think about exactly what your anxiety has cost you in the past and what it's costing you today.

Are you willing to continue to pay that price, or like Whitney and Lena, are you ready to start making some changes?

If you are ready to make some changes, let's agree to work together to assemble an anxiety-busting tool kit you can use to help you face your fears. Let's create a plan for easing your anxiety and helping you step back into life. And let's begin by taking a closer look at exactly how your anxiety shows up in your life.

CHAPTER 5

A Checklist of *Your* Anxiety Symptoms

DOES YOUR anxiety show up in your life inwardly, in your emotions or your thinking, or does it show up outwardly, in your physical body?

If you're not sure, completing the following checklist will give you more information about how you experience anxiety. Just put a check beside any answer that is true for you.

_____   1. I feel shaky.
_____   2. I find it difficult to concentrate. Sometimes my thoughts race and/or sometimes my mind goes blank.
_____   3. My stomach is upset (I'm constipated, I have diarrhea, or I'm nauseous).
_____   4. I feel detached from reality.
_____   5. I get sweaty even when it's not hot.
_____   6. I'm afraid I'm losing my mind.
_____   7. My heart pounds. I have palpitations or I breathe rapidly.

_____ 8. I feel detached from my body.

_____ 9. I have pain and/or pressure in my chest.

_____ 10. I worry things will never get better.

_____ 11. I have trouble swallowing.

_____ 12. I have panic attacks.

_____ 13. I have unexplained hot and/or cold flashes.

_____ 14. I worry about getting sick, having a heart attack, or dying.

_____ 15. I have dizzy spells and sometimes feel like I'm going to faint.

_____ 16. I'm terrified that something terrible is going to happen.

_____ 17. I'm tired all the time, even after a good night's sleep.

_____ 18. I fear looking stupid or inadequate.

_____ 19. I get headaches.

_____ 20. I dread the thought of leaving home or trying something new.

_____ 21. I can't relax my body, no matter how hard I try.

_____ 22. I'm afraid of being alone.

_____ 23. My toes and/or fingers are tingling.

_____ 24. I worry 24/7, sometimes about nothing at all.

_____ 25. My mouth is dry.

_____ 26. I'm afraid of facing an object (like a snake or a spider) or a situation (like flying or speaking in public).

_____ 27. I often feel like I'm going to cry.

_____ 28. I dread social situations.

_____ 29. My muscles are unusually tense.

_____ 30. I'm irritable and/or have outbursts of anger.

What the Numbers Mean

Now that you've finished the checklist, let's get specific about what all these numbers mean to you and your anxiety.

First count up the number of checkmarks you put beside the even numbers and put that number here:

Now count up the number of checkmarks beside the odd numbers and put that number here:

Did you check off more even numbers or more odd numbers?

If you checked off more odd numbers, that means your anxiety tends to show up mainly in your body. And the more even numbers you've checked, the more your anxiety tends to show up in physical symptoms. It also means you're not alone. A majority of women report having physical symptoms of anxiety—especially symptoms like headaches, an upset stomach, or the feeling of wanting to cry.

If you've checked off more even numbers, that means your anxiety is an inside job, showing up in your thoughts and emotions. And the more odd numbers you've checked off, the more your anxiety is likely to manifest in some negative thinking.

So how does anxiety show up for you—physically or mentally?

CHAPTER 6

Where to Start

That the birds of worry and care fly over your head,

this you cannot change, but that they build nests

in your hair, this you can prevent.

—Chinese proverb

NOW THAT you know more about how your anxiety shows up in your life, you have an important clue about the best way for you to start *your* healing process. In *Yoga as Medicine*, Timothy McCall describes a study done by Dr. Jon Kabat-Zinn, founder of the stress-reduction clinic at the University of Massachusetts. Kabat-Zinn reports that "patients whose anxiety manifested mainly in mental symptoms like constant worrying tended to find hatha yoga preferable to mindfulness meditation, whereas those whose symptoms of anxiety tended to manifest mainly in the body preferred the less body-oriented meditation.

"As Kabat-Zinn says, 'People need different doors to come into the room, so to speak, of self-awareness and self-knowing. Some people just can't go through the mind door. They get the body door instantly.' For others the opposite is true."

So what does this all mean for you? It means there's more than one way to heal anxiety. You can use physical tools like qigong, yoga, acupressure, massage, dancing, laughing, deep breathing, et cetera. Or you can employ mental techniques like affirmations, reframing, meditation, asking better questions, etc.

But Kabat-Zinn's research gives you a clue about what might be the easiest place for *you* to start. When anxiety shows up in the *body*, working with the tools that use your *mind* might be more effective for you. You may want to turn first to the chapters on meditation, CBT, or "The Work."

But if you checked off more even numbers, your anxiety is showing up in your thoughts and emotions. You may want to consider starting with the more physical approaches like yoga, qigong, or just going for a walk.

As always, do what's right for you. When you're not sure, when you feel lost, stop. Listen to your body, your mind, and your emotions. Just like that GPS in your phone or car, they will guide you to a peaceful new way of being. Start where you need to start. Take out a tool or two and give it a try. If something doesn't work, that's okay. Try something else, and keep on trying until you find the things that bring you comfort and ease.

PART TWO

CLAIM YOUR ANXIETY

Claiming your power is an inside job.

—Author unknown

CHAPTER 7

How to Claim
Your Anxiety

Begin challenging your own assumptions.
Your assumptions are the windows on the world.
Scrub them off every once in a while, or the light won't come in.

—Alan Alda, actor, director, and author of *If I Understood You,*
Would I Have This Look on My Face?

ERE'S THE most powerful thing I've learned about anxiety in all my years of dealing with it, studying it, and cursing it. This is the absolute truth about my anxiety and yours, and it's the best and worst news possible.

So get ready. Take a deep breath and fasten your seat belt, because this is going to change everything: your thinking, your willingness to take action, and finally your life.

You are causing your anxiety.

It may not feel like it, but the worrying you do and the thoughts that keep you up at night and make you afraid to leave your home in the morning are all your own creation. You are making yourself afraid.

Let me say it another way. Worry is all an inside job and it's inside *you*.

Now, you may be arguing, "You don't know my boss." "You don't know my partner, my parents, my health. Anyone with a child in such trouble would be waking up at night in a sweat. Anyone with my diagnosis . . . my physical challenges . . . my *life* would feel exactly the way I do."

I hear you. I've done my share of waiting for the results of medical tests. I've battled cancer twice, lost a baby, raised children, cared for an aging parent, worried about car payments, and worked crazy hours at challenging jobs. I know what it's like to stare at the ceiling at 3:00 a.m., heart thundering, mind racing.

But let me say it again: You are causing your own anxiety.

No matter what happens to you, you get to choose:

1. How you think about it
2. How you feel about it
3. And what you're going to do about it

I promise you, there isn't a person, place, or thing in this world that can make you anxious without your permission. Your mother, brother, partner, or boss cannot make you anxious unless you allow them to. The government, your teachers, your coworkers—even the weather—can't force you to be anxious.

I know it may be hard to believe that a wonderfully talented, smart woman like you could be causing yourself such misery. But it's the *truth*. And when you embrace that truth, acknowledge your own incredible power, and start choosing to think differently, you will be in charge of your anxiety for once and always. Now, I call that GOOD NEWS.

You don't have to rely on someone or something else to change. You don't have to wait for someone else to soothe your pain or set you free from the prison of your fears. You can do it for yourself. All you have to do is work with me to create a tool kit of techniques and ideas to help you shift the way you think, feel, and act.

So it's simple, right?

Well, not really.

Changing the way you think about the world is a long-term, complicated process that, in my experience, requires patience, a gentle caring for your spirit, and a willingness to think about things in a new way.

But you can begin to experience the power of change in this moment by saying to yourself, "I'm ready to try something different. I am ready to change the way I think about myself and my life. I am ready to let go of this fear."

Here's a visualization exercise to help you start releasing your fear. I suggest you read it through a few times to get the idea of how this works before giving it a try.

Dissolving Anxiety

Begin by letting your breath deepen as you settle more comfortably in your chair. Close your eyes. As you continue to breathe even more deeply, let your belly soften. Let your shoulders relax. Loosen your jaw and let the tension drain from your body. Feel yourself sink into the chair, knowing it will support your weight. Know that you are safe in this moment. There's nowhere else you need to be, nothing else you should be doing. This moment is for you.

Now, imagine your fear is a heavy black rock that exists somewhere in your body. Maybe it's in your chest or your belly. Take a moment to find it inside you. Once you've located it, notice its size and weight. Notice how much space it takes inside you and how it weighs you down. Feel how it limits your ability to live and move and breathe. Feel how it presses you into your chair, making the smallest motion difficult.

As you continue to breathe, put your hands over the part of your body where you feel that rock. Take a moment to notice what it feels like.

Now, imagine your hands begin to grow warm and radiate a beautiful silver light that flows through your hands into your body. Know that light has the power to dissolve the rock within you as easily as hot water melts ice. Imagine feeling the rock slowly melting away, draining out of your body and into the ground below, leaving a lovely place of ease and calm inside you. As the last of that rock fades away, feel the lightness of your body. Feel the sense of freedom that follows.

Take a moment to enjoy that sense of freedom, that amazing core of calm inside. Put your hands over your heart and just breathe as you slowly allow yourself to come back to full consciousness. Now take that sense of calm and peace with you into your day.

You can do this exercise a hundred times a day. The more you do it, the better you'll feel and the more peaceful your life will become.

Now that we've taken this first step to easing your anxiety, let's take a closer look at exactly when, where, and how that anxiety shows up in your life.

CHAPTER 8

Logging In

The key is not to prioritize what's on your schedule,
but to schedule your priorities.

—Stephen Covey, businessman and author of
The 7 Habits of Highly Effective People

THE BEST way I've found to really get to know your anxiety is to keep a log of your thoughts and feelings for a few days. This may sound like a lot of work, but taking an hour-by-hour look at when and where anxiety pops up in your life allows you to see what's triggering your anxiety, as well as patterns of behavior, thoughts, and emotions. It can also highlight the particular "ins and outs" of *your* anxiety.

Make It Your Own

You can keep your daily log by using a regular calendar, a journal, or your phone, or you can keep track online. You can create your own log by using the template in this book as an example, or you can come up with your own design.

You can make your entries as you go through your day. (This is the most effective approach because the data is fresh in your mind, but it isn't always possible.) Or you can log in at mealtime or before bed as a way to review the day. Do what works best for you. But do it. Getting to know *who* and *where* you are today is the first step on the journey to where you want to be tomorrow.

Let's take a look at how Gloria found keeping a log helped her deal with the stress and worry of retirement.

Gloria and her husband had been planning for years to retire to a warmer climate. At sixty-five, Gloria was thrilled to finally be able to leave her job as an office manager, sell the home where they'd raised their three sons, and move south to a beautiful new house.

Gloria believed she was at last going to get to live the life of ease and joy she'd been longing for. But instead she was blindsided by sudden episodes of anxiety and panic that seemed to come from out of nowhere.

When talking to Ellen, her longtime work friend, Gloria explained, "I've always been a little anxious, but without my usual routine, my job, my friends, and my old house, I feel like I don't know who I am anymore. I feel overwhelmed and anxious, and I don't know what to do about it."

Ellen suggested she try the tracking technique they'd used in the office to get a better look at a problem they were wrestling with.

Gloria decided to keep track in a journal she designed herself. She wrote in her log every evening after dinner and kept her answers simple. Within a few days, she noticed she was most anxious in the morning as she was getting ready for the day ahead. She also noticed she had almost no anxiety on days when she'd made plans ahead of time or had something to look forward to, like a Zoom call with her grandchildren. She also did better on days when she ate her meals at regular times.

As she studied her daily log, Gloria decided that she needed to bring some structure to her days. She needed to plan things to do ahead of time and to include things she would look forward to doing.

Gloria began scheduling meals at the same time every day. She signed up for a class in archaeology and one in tai chi. She scheduled at least one call with every grandchild every week, and she and her husband began planning the trip to Asia she'd always wanted to take.

As she made these changes, Gloria began to view retirement not as a dead end, but as an opportunity to explore things she loved and spend time with family and new friends.

A few months later, when talking to Ellen, Gloria was able to tell her that retirement was everything she'd hoped it would be.

So why not try keeping a log for the next few days and see what comes up for you?

The following Daily Anxiety Log is a suggestion of one way you could keep track. Use it to get you started with the process or in any way that works for you.

Daily Anxiety Log

Date: _____

TIME	WHAT I'M DOING (ACTIVITY/ SITUATION)	WHAT I'M TELLING MYSELF	ANXIETY LEVEL (1–10)*
12:00 a.m.			
1:00 a.m.			
2:00 a.m.			
3:00 a.m.			
4:00 a.m.			
5:00 a.m.			
6:00 a.m.			
7:00 a.m.			
8:00 a.m.			
9:00 a.m.			
10:00 a.m.			
11:00 a.m.			
12:00 p.m.			
1:00 p.m.			
2:00 p.m.			
3:00 p.m.			
4:00 p.m.			
5:00 p.m.			
6:00 p.m.			
7:00 p.m.			
8:00 p.m.			
9:00 p.m.			
10:00 p.m.			
11:00 p.m.			

* (Anxiety level 1 = complete calm; anxiety level 10 = panic attack)

Reviewing the Data

As you read over your anxiety log, be on the lookout for triggers, patterns, and cycles. Also, here are some questions you might want to keep in mind to help bring clarity to the process:

1. When am I anxious? How often? Once a day? Twice a day? More than that?
2. *What* or *who* makes me anxious?
3. What *thoughts* make me anxious?
4. Is there something that *always* triggers my anxiety?
5. Can I predict my anxiety, or does it seem to come from nowhere?
6. How long does my anxiety last?
7. Are there times during the day when I'm not anxious at all?
8. How much sleep am I getting? When and what am I eating?
9. Where am I in my monthly cycle? Does that make a difference?
10. Were there times in the past I successfully managed my anxiety? How?
11. What have I done to cope with my anxiety that did *not* work?
12. Does keeping track of my anxiety make a difference in how I feel? Has it changed the way I feel about my anxiety?

As Suze Orman, financial expert and author of *The 9 Steps to Financial Freedom*, says so well, "It's impossible to map out a route to your destination if you don't know where you're starting from."

This is a great place to start creating your brave, new life.

CHAPTER 9

When to Get Help

If you break your knee, you have therapy,
and it's the same for your heart.

—Toni Braxton, singer and songwriter, best known for
"Un-Break My Heart" and "You Mean the World to Me"

AROUND MY house we have lots of discussions about what repairs and chores we can handle ourselves and when we need to "call for help." Sometimes it's really clear that changing the filter is something we can manage on our own. It's equally clear that we're going to need an expert to deal with the water dripping from the light fixture on the kitchen ceiling.

Deciding when to seek professional help for your anxiety is a similar process. Is this something you can take care of yourself by talking to friends or reading a few good books, or do you need to call for help?

If you're thinking maybe you could use some professional help, here are two questions to ask yourself.

1. Does the issue I'm dealing with affect my life in a major way? If not, maybe this is something you can deal with yourself.
2. Am I suffering in silence? If you're suffering in any way, it's time to reach out and get help. If you'd broken your arm or were experiencing chest pains, you'd ask for help. Same here. Promise me—*no more suffering*.

If you're still on the fence about getting help, here are some guidelines to help you sort through your challenges and choices.

Suicidal thoughts or plans. If you're seriously thinking about killing yourself, if you have a plan to kill yourself or harm yourself in any way, please put down this book and go call for help. NOW!

- Call a trusted friend.
- Call 911.
- Go to the nearest emergency room.
- Call the National Suicide Prevention Lifeline at 1-800-273-TALK (8255).
- Visit http://www.suicidepreventionlifeline.org/.

Please don't hesitate. Stop living in pain. Reach out for help. Tell the truth about what's going on with you. No matter how hopeless things feel right now, there is help for you, I promise. But no one can help you until you take this first step. Go ahead. Help is on the other end of that line.

Trauma. If you've experienced a traumatic event and are having trouble sleeping, suffering from flashbacks, nightmares, depression, or anxiety, or experiencing any other lingering side effects of that trauma, you may want to consider getting professional help.

Maybe you feel you're "doing okay." Nobody would guess from looking at you or your life that you're a mess inside. But "doing okay" is not good enough. And getting help will get you started on the road to feeling better.

Grief. The same things that are true about trauma are true about grief. Loss and grief are a part of life. But if your grief isn't better after six to twelve months and it's interfering with your life, seeking help can be useful in getting back to the joy of living. Stop suffering. Start living.

Feeling hopeless. If you're feeling hopeless, if you're telling yourself that nothing's ever going to change and there's no joy left in your life, therapy can help you find hope again. If you've lost interest in the things you used to love to do, if you're feeling like this is *never* going to get better, then getting help can bring back your sense of perspective and maybe even allow you to find the fun again.

Drug/alcohol abuse and other addictions. If you're turning to a substance or have an addiction to anything that affects the quality of your life—for instance, gambling, sex, shopping, or overeating—then getting treatment can help you deal with that abuse/addiction and get your life back on track.

Your life isn't working anymore. You're sad. You're scared. Things around you are out of control. You walk around feeling angry at the world for no particular reason (or for some very particular reason). Somehow you've run your life into a ditch. Nothing's getting better and you don't know what the heck to do. Getting some help can often turn these life challenges around. So make a call and get started feeling better soon.

Physical symptoms. You've been to your PCP. She's done all the tests and can't find anything wrong with you physically. Maybe that stomachache, sore neck, sleeplessness, tight jaw, or headache is a symptom of something going on with you emotionally. Going to a professional may provide you with some answers as to what's going on with you physically and can help you find ways to heal your mind and your body.

Advice from others. Someone close to you suggests that you should get some help. I suggest you swallow hard, say "thank you," and consider their suggestion. They may be right.

A difficult change. There's been a change in your life and you're not handling it well. You've recently divorced, been diagnosed, moved to a new state, lost your job, got a job, had a baby, adopted a child, or retired. There are all sorts of changes that happen to us throughout our lives. Some are expected and some are a real surprise.

Whether the change is something you've worked hard to bring about or it happens out of the blue, change can really upset the balance of your life. If you're having trouble coping with a change, talking to someone can help you restore balance and calm to your life.

Realizing you can't do it alone. One morning you wake up thinking, "I'm tired of doing this alone. What I'm doing isn't working." Maybe, like me, you've been reading all the books and struggling along on your own. If you feel like you've been battling anxiety on your own and not making progress, talking to a professional might get you back on the road to feeling good again.

Finally, therapy doesn't have to be a lifetime commitment. David Sack, MD, reports in a study published in the *Journal of Consulting and Clinical Psychology* that "88 percent of therapy-goers reported improvements after just one session."

Let me repeat that good news. *After just one therapy session, 88 percent of clients felt better.*

So now that you're considering getting some professional help, how exactly do you go about getting the right help for you?

Turn the page to read more about how to hire a professional who best fits your needs.

CHAPTER 10

How to Get Help

I wish more people would talk about therapy.
We girls, we're taught to be almost too resilient,
to be strong and sexy and cool and laid-back, the girl
who's down. We also need to feel allowed to fall apart.

—Selena Gomez, singer, songwriter, and actress

Getting Started

How do you go about finding the therapist that's right for you? According to an article in *Consumer Reports*, studies show that "people who find a therapist through a recommendation from a friend, family member, or doctor have more success than those who pick someone at random from the phone book or their health plan's provider directory."

If you're hesitant about asking friends or family or don't have a primary care physician, you can call a local university with a good psychology department and ask for a recommendation. Or you can get in touch with a professional organization that has screened their members and will stand behind them.

Here are some you might try:

- The American Psychological Association
- *Psychology Today*
- The Association for Behavioral and Cognitive Therapies
- Anxiety and Depression Association of America

Questions to Ask a Potential Therapist

Before you sit down with a therapist, it's important to know what to expect from the process. Here are some questions you can ask to get the conversation started.

1. Are you licensed and/or credentialed?
2. How long have you been in practice?
3. Are you accepting new clients?
4. Do you have a specialty (anxiety, depression, OCD)?
5. What kinds of treatments do you offer? What treatments would you use for someone with my diagnosis?
6. Where are you located?
7. When are you available? What happens in case I have an emergency?
8. How long do you think treatment might take?
9. Does my insurance cover your services? Will I have a copay?
10. If my insurance doesn't cover your services, do you offer a sliding scale?

As you chat with the therapist, look for a connection. Does she answer your questions in a way that makes sense? Do you feel comfortable with her? If not, this isn't the therapist for you. The bond between client and therapist is essential to the process of healing.

> If cost is an issue for you, you may be able to find afforda-
> ble mental health care through the Substance Abuse and
> Mental Health Services Administration at http://www.
> samhsa.gov/treatment or call 1-800-662-HELP (4357).

Stigma

The good news for women is that we're far more likely than men to seek professional help for our anxiety. The less good news is that there's still a stigma attached to anyone seeking mental health care. Women who wouldn't think twice about going to the doctor with the flu or a UTI hesitate at the idea of going for therapy.

We whisper about poor Hezzie who couldn't handle that divorce on her own and had to go "see somebody." We tell one another we can't afford therapy or it's only for losers and crazy people, not smart, tough women like us.

Or we're so ashamed of the abuse, the addiction, or the secret we're keeping that the last thing we want to do is share that weakness with another human being.

There are literally hundreds of reasons women put off going for therapy, but here's the truth.

Most people who seek therapy aren't crazy. They're not broken, bad, friendless, or weak. They're people like you and me who need a little help in dealing with their lives. So if you're suffering with anxiety as you read this, please reach out for help. You don't have to do this alone.

And if you're too uncomfortable at the thought of talking to a stranger in person, or there isn't a therapist in your area, you can now get therapy online.

Finally, remember you are the customer. You and/or your insurance company are paying for the service. If, for any reason, you aren't happy with the way things are going, speak up. Let the professional know what's not working for you about the relationship, the fees, or the service in general. It may be awkward to bring up the subject of money or the fact that the therapist is never on time or seems distracted during your session, but if you don't bring it up, it won't get fixed.

I think there's a lot of confusion about who does what in the mental health profession. This chart will give you some idea of how best to get your needs met if you decide to seek help.

Who's Who in Mental Health

TITLE	TALK THERAPY	MEDICATION
Psychiatrist	Depends on the state	Yes
Psychologist	Yes	Depends on the state
Psychiatric Mental Health Nurse	Yes	Yes
Licensed Social Worker	Yes	No
Licensed Professional Counselor	Yes	No

PART THREE

REFRAME YOUR ANXIETY

You must master a new way to think before you can master a new way to be.

—Marianne Williamson,
American spiritual guide and author

CHAPTER 11

Beck's Anxiety Equation

Anxiety = Uncertainty × Powerlessness

—Chip Conley, entrepreneur and author of *Emotional Equations*

THE FIRST time I saw Beck's anxiety equation was truly an "aha!" moment for me. At one glance, I saw exactly how I was creating my own anxiety. My thoughts and beliefs were the only things making me so anxious. And I realized that if I could make myself afraid with my thoughts, I could change those thoughts and literally think myself out of those debilitating feelings of fear and panic. Wow!

Aaron Beck, an American psychiatrist, has been called "the father of cognitive therapy." If you go see a licensed therapist, chances are she's been influenced by Beck's work. For me, his equation brought clarity and insight to a subject that had seemed complicated and confusing. I hope it does the same for you.

Now, if you're a numbers person, please know that Beck saw this quasi-equation as a way to *describe* anxiety, not measure it. If you're not a numbers person, please don't skip this part because you think it will be too complicated to understand. Stick with me on this. You'll be glad you did.

So, here is Beck's equation:

$$Anxiety = \frac{Perceived\ Probability\ of\ Threat \times Perceived\ Cost\ of\ Threat}{Perceived\ Ability\ to\ Cope \times Perceived\ Rescue\ Factors}$$

In other words, anxiety is the result of an imbalance between the perceived threat and your perceived ability to cope with that threat. Again, don't worry if this still seems confusing. We're going to spend some time looking at this equation more closely.

The Factors Above the Line:
Perceived Probability of Threat × Perceived Cost of Threat

Perceived Probability of Threat

The more likely you think it is that the danger could actually happen, the more anxious you'll be.

If Erin absolutely believes the earth is going to be hit by an asteroid next Tuesday, then that belief is going to raise her anxiety level sky-high. If, on the other hand, she's not sure about the asteroid thing, the threat and her fear will automatically be lower.

Perceived Cost of Threat

The more miserable you believe this threat could make you, the more anxious you're going to be about it.

If Agnes believes the little spider in her bedroom is poisonous and one bite will kill her, I bet she's going to be a lot more anxious than if she believes that the spider is harmless. See the difference?

The Factors Below the Line:
Perceived Ability to Cope × Perceived Rescue Factors

Perceived Ability to Cope

How well do you think you're going to be able to deal with all those dangers lurking above the line? If you feel capable and strong, those dangers may not seem so scary. If you feel lost, tired, or too afraid to take action, those dangers will look bigger and much more terrifying.

Take a moment to think about how you'd rate your confidence level in general. Do you wake up every morning knowing you're not going to be able to meet your quotas at work? Are you sure you're never going to be able to find the right gift to bring to the shower or cook a dinner that pleases everyone in your family? Guess what's probably going to happen.

Or do you tell yourself you can always count on yourself to do your best? Do you remind yourself that everyone deserves a great life, especially you?

Can you feel the difference between those two beliefs? Which one do you think serves you better?

Perceived Rescue Factors

How likely is it that someone or something else is going to come along and rescue you? If Clara believes she has a friend in her corner who will help her no matter what, how do you think she would feel about going back to law school in her forties? Do you think the belief that she could always call on a higher power in any situation would make a difference in how she thought about and handled stress?

How about you? If you knew you could always rely on a helping hand to get you through whatever lies ahead, do you think that would affect your anxiety level?

Hmm . . .

So now that we've taken a look at Beck's equation, let's take a look at how that equation can change the way you think and feel about your anxiety.

CHAPTER 12

What I Think Is Making Me Anxious (Cognitive Behavioral Therapy)

When you change the way you look at things,
the things you look at change.

—Wayne Dyer, psychologist and author of *Change Your Thoughts—*
Change Your Life and Your Erroneous Zones

AS A cognitive behavioral therapist, here's what I believe about the way we think. (There are lots of other approaches to therapy and thoughts about thinking. This is what works for *me*.) What you *think* about something creates your emotional reaction to it. And that emotional reaction causes you to take action. In other words, your thoughts, opinions, and/or beliefs are the driving force in how you feel about the world and how you react to life.

For instance, Tina was bitten by a dog when she was eight. Her reaction to an approaching Boston terrier might be:

1. Her thinking: Oh my God, it's a DOG. They're dangerous animals.
2. Her emotional reaction: I'm afraid.
3. Her action: Run.

On the other hand, Chloe grew up in a home that took in foster dogs. Her reaction to the approach of the same Boston terrier might be:

1. Her thinking: Oh good, it's a DOG. They're wonderful animals.
2. Her emotional reaction: I'm excited.
3. Her action: Approach. Pat the dog.

If our thoughts are the source of *all* our emotions, including anxiety, it stands to reason that if we changed our thoughts, our emotions would change. And if we *felt* differently about things, we would *act* differently. It's that simple. If you change your thinking, your anxiety will ease and your life will change.

All right, maybe it's really not that simple.

If you've already tried changing your thoughts and beliefs, you may have noticed how quickly thoughts come and go in our brains and how many of those thoughts are negative.

Beck calls those thoughts automatic negative thoughts (ANTS), and that's exactly what they seem to be, automatic responses to the outer world. It may seem to you that those thoughts come and go on their own, but I promise you, you are choosing to think those thoughts.

These thoughts are *learned responses*. They may have come from your parents, your seventh-grade math teacher, or a kid on the playground. "Don't eat that." "Don't touch that." "Shame on you." "You're not good at science." "You're just a girl." "You're never going to amount to anything." "You don't deserve to succeed." "The world is a scary, unsafe place and you're not going to be able to handle the terrible things that are going to happen to you, so don't even try."

Those thoughts may also be the result of past experiences, especially trauma. The time you got up to speak and your mind went blank, the day you dropped the ball in the big game, the afternoon you were in that terrible accident.

These thoughts began as a one-time entry into your computer brain, but for one reason or another, they had enough power and importance for you to choose to think them again and again. "I'm not good at fixing things." "I'm not like everyone else." "Cars are dangerous."

It's no longer a one-time thought, but a thought that loops over and over in your brain. And as that thought continually passes through your brain, it creates a worn, familiar pathway that allows it to travel that way ever more easily until, without you being aware of it, it becomes a part of you and your response to the world.

Some of these thoughts and beliefs are helpful and serve you well. "Check your rearview mirror before backing up." "Don't hike alone in the woods." "Bring an umbrella."

But some of these automatic negative thoughts are worse than useless. They're judgmental and mean, and they may be the very thing that's keeping you stuck and afraid. And here's the kicker. *These sneaky thoughts are running your life and you may not have even been aware of them.* Until now.

So, let's take the first step and identify some of those unhealthy, irrational thoughts.

According to Albert Ellis, creator of REBT (Rational Emotive Behavior Therapy), there are twelve major irrational beliefs.

As you read this list of the twelve irrational beliefs, be on the lookout for the ones that resonate with you and circle them. Can you remember the first time you thought those thoughts? Did your mom believe it? Your dad? Does your belief come from a negative experience? Observation? The more you know about these hidden beliefs, the better you'll be at recognizing and changing them.

Ellis's Twelve Irrational Beliefs

1. Everyone must love me. God help me if someone disapproves of the way I look, sound, dance, or breathe. God help us all if I can't make them *all* love me. That's my job!

Do you recognize any part of the first irrational belief in your own thinking? What if you decided to just please yourself, instead of everyone around you?

2. I must always be perfect. I must always be incredibly successful at everything I do. Failure is not an option.

Do you recognize any part of the second irrational belief in your own thinking? What do you think would *really* happen if you failed? What if you knew you could handle even the worst possible outcome?

3. Everyone else has to be perfect, too. If the people around me fall short of my standards, I must judge them harshly. They must be blamed and punished.

Do you recognize any part of the third irrational belief in your own thinking? What if you started believing that everyone was doing their best? (Not that their best was good or right, just that they did the best they could at the time.)

4. I want what I want. Everything has to go my way. If it doesn't, I'll hold my breath until I turn blue.

Do you recognize any part of the fourth irrational belief in your own thinking? What if everything was all right just the way it was?

5. I have no control over the way I feel. It's *their* fault I feel this way. It's the government, the weather, my parents, and/or that cranky neighbor that's making me miserable.

Do you recognize any part of the fifth irrational belief in your own thinking? How would you feel if you could control your emotions by changing your thinking?

6. If I think long and hard enough about this possible disaster, disease, danger, or crisis, it won't happen. I'm so powerful I can protect myself and my loved ones with just my thoughts.

Do you recognize any part of the sixth irrational belief in your own thinking? What if you told yourself that no matter what happened, you'd be able to handle it?

7. My life will be easier if I just hide under my bed and ignore the unpleasant, scary commitments, conversations, difficult tasks, or circumstances that show up in my life. I'll be all right if I just pretend nothing is happening. If I don't acknowledge it, it can't hurt me.

Do you recognize any part of the seventh irrational belief in your own thinking? What if you could break that task into manageable little bits? What if you focused on how you'll feel after you've finished the task? What if you asked for help?

8. I'll never be able do anything worthwhile by myself. I can't do this. I'm going to have to depend on someone smarter or more capable to take care of it for me.

Do you recognize any part of the eighth irrational belief in your own thinking? What if you decided you could depend on *you*? What if you started today to take care of yourself?

9. My past always determines my present. Events in my past (childhood included) have made and always will make me anxious and miserable. I cannot escape my history.

Do you recognize any part of the ninth irrational belief in your own thinking? What if you decided to retell the story you tell yourself about your past in a way that changes it into a story of power and success? What if you chose to forgive yourself and everyone else for what happened and gave yourself a chance to start anew?

10. I should suffer as much or more over the problems and challenges of my friends and family as they do. If they're not worried enough, I have to take on that worry for them. Really, do I have to do everything myself?

Do you recognize any part of the tenth irrational belief in your own thinking? What if you allowed the people around you to claim their own strength and resolve as they solve their own problems?

11. There is only one perfect solution to every problem. I must find it or face the consequences. I have to do this right. There's no margin for error. Failure is not an option.

Do you recognize any part of the eleventh irrational belief in your own thinking? What if you could come up with a couple of possible solutions, then picked the best of the bunch?

12. I must judge myself and everyone else on the planet with my own harsh rating scale. I have very high standards and it's my job to make sure everyone meets them. And I take that job very seriously.

Do you recognize any part of the twelfth irrational belief in your own thinking? What if you decided to believe that people, including you, are always doing the best they can?

There you have Ellis's top-twelve irrational beliefs. I've come up with some of my own over the years, including:

1. If I do well, everyone will hate me. I have to hide my success.
2. There is never enough to go around. If someone else succeeds, they're taking my stuff.

Are there any of yours that we've missed? Are there some other irrational ideas that are holding you hostage? Write them here:

1.

2.

3.

Once you identify the automatic thoughts that run your life, you can begin to release, change, or rethink the ones that don't work.

But it's not just the *thoughts* we're thinking that get us into trouble. The *way* we think can be just as troublesome.

So let's take a look at some more stinking thinking.

CHAPTER 13

How I Think Is Making Me Anxious, Too (More Cognitive Behavioral Therapy)

Whether you think you can, or you
think you can't, you're right.

—Henry Ford, industrialist and business magnate,
author of *My Life and Work*

I T'S NOT just what you think that can make you anxious. *How* you think can make you just as miserable. The following ten "cognitive distortions" or, in plain English, "ten screwed-up ways we think" come from *The Feeling Good Handbook* by David Burns.

As you read through them, see how many apply to you. Odds are you've experienced most of them at some time in your life, but what

69

we're looking for here is a *consistent pattern of thinking that does not work for you*. As always, if what you're doing is working, keep right on doing it. But if you find you're anxious, depressed, confused, or just plain pissed off, maybe it's the *way* you're thinking that's making you feel so crummy.

So let's get started.

1. All-or-nothing thinking: You're either right or you're wrong. There is no gray area for you. Hope is trying to lose weight but finds herself either eating nothing but broccoli and grapefruit or living on pecan pie, pizza, and chocolate gelato. There's no place in between for her. Either she does the job perfectly or not at all. There's no forgiveness, no middle ground. There are two choices, good and bad. Period.

Do you recognize any part of this first cognitive distortion? What if you could allow yourself to imagine what new ideas might be in the gray area?

2. Overgeneralization: One past mistake or traumatic event convinces you that you're a complete loser, doomed to endure tragedy for the rest of your life. Oh, the drama of it all. If you messed up your first marriage, got fired from your last job, or failed math in the seventh grade, you're doomed to die alone, never get another good job, and not figure out the tip at dinner. When Karen's father left her mother, Karen decided all marriages were doomed to fail—so why even date? She was never going to get married and go through that pain. No way.

Do you recognize any part of this second cognitive distortion? What if you allowed yourself to believe that what you did in the past is over and you can choose a new beginning anytime you want? What if this is that moment you change everything?

3. Mental filter: You focus fiercely on the worst of any situation and ignore the positives. Sharissa rented a new apartment. It was perfect except that the bathroom was an ugly shade of khaki green. So what did she focus on? What did she talk about? Right, the hideous color. Ruth loves her partner, Jodie, but Jodie's really messy. Ruth is so focused on that messiness that she misses Jodie's generous spirit and heart, and that focus puts their relationship in jeopardy.

Do you recognize any part of this third cognitive distortion? What if you could change your focus for just an instant to what is working for you? Go ahead. Give it a try. What if you did that more often?

4. *Discounting the positives*: Jada could talk about her failures and mistakes at length. Yet she looked confused and uncertain when asked to talk about her strengths and successes. She said things like, "Of course I'm good at my job. Isn't everyone?" "I enjoy teaching sign language in my spare time, but it's no big deal." "The award I won last year really doesn't count."

How about *you*? Do you discount your strengths? Do you recognize any part of this fourth cognitive distortion? What if you celebrated your successes instead of discounting them? What if you focused on your strengths for a change? (See "Accentuate the Positive," p. 114.)

5. *Jumping to conclusions*: Rosanna could see the future and knew it was going to be awful. She believed she could read people's minds and they didn't like her. With no proof at all, she knew her next quarter was going to stink and that cough was much more serious than it sounded. She didn't have to ask the man she'd just started seeing how he felt—she knew he was planning to dump her. Talk about snatching defeat from the jaws of victory.

Do you recognize any part of this fifth cognitive distortion? What if you used that wonderful magical ability to imagine a positive future and the best in the people around you?

6. *Magnification or minimization*: More drama here. Fran was prepared for disaster to strike at any moment. She had an uncanny ability to see the worst in any situation and instantly make it more awful. For instance, when her husband was ten minutes late getting home and hadn't called, Fran decided he'd been in a terrible car crash. She imagined him strapped to a stretcher in the back of an ambulance hurtling toward an emergency room. What if he didn't survive?

How would Fran get through the funeral? How would she keep the house on just her salary? How would she meet anyone else? She was doomed to die alone.

See how it works? The more creative you are, the more miserable you can make yourself. The other side of this is that you minimize your competence and abilities until you convince yourself you'll never be able to cope with what life throws at you.

Do you recognize any part of this sixth cognitive distortion? What if you just started telling yourself the truth?

7. *Emotional reasoning*: Betty believed her emotions were the truth, instead of the other way around. Her feelings of guilt caused her to believe she'd done something wrong even when she hadn't. Fiona was terrified of speaking in public, so she decided that meant that giving a speech is a very risky thing to do and avoided it at all costs.

This seventh distortion is sneaky and can have been a part of your life for such a long time it's hard to spot. In order to root out emotional reasoning, you may want to challenge the validity of your perceptions of both yourself and the world around you. Is what you believe true, or are your emotions making you believe it's true? (See "A Reframe of Reframing," p. 80.)

Do you recognize any part of this seventh cognitive distortion? What would you like to believe instead?

8. *"Should" statements*: Boy, this is a tough one, and probably the most common. It's about the expectations you have for your-self and others, as well as the expectations they have for you. (You can substitute here the words "must," "have to," or "need to," as well as "shouldn't," "mustn't," "don't have to," "don't need to," etc.) "I should look better." "I should feel better." "I should be on time." "I should make more money, lose weight. I should be less anxious." "They should be nicer, take better care of me, stop saying those mean things." "My sister should show up on time."

Albert Ellis said stop "shoulding" on yourself. I agree. No "shoulding" on you or on others.

Do you recognize any part of this eighth cognitive distortion? What if you struck the word "should" from your vocabulary and said "choose to" instead?

9. *Labeling*: Now, instead of just recognizing your failings and moving on, you stop and give them a whole new importance by naming them. When Eve did poorly on a test, she didn't give herself credit for studying hard or doing her best. She turned the spotlight on her shortcomings and called herself names like "stupid" and "hopeless." When others let her down, she did the same to them, labeling them as "greedy," or "mean," or "evil."

Do you recognize any part of this ninth cognitive distortion? What if you agreed to stop naming your failures and the failures of others? What if you forgave yourself/others and just moved on?

10. *Personalization and blame*: You take the blame for something that isn't your fault. Winona was thrilled to land a job at a new company. But three weeks later, the company went out of business and she blamed herself. She decided that hiring her was the reason they'd failed. Her incompetence was what put them in bankruptcy. Debra blamed everyone else for the drama in her life. *It's my mother's fault that I'm not getting ahead. It's my son's fault I don't have time to get my laundry done, so I'm wearing this blouse for the third time this week.*

Really?

Do you recognize any part of this tenth cognitive distortion? What if you didn't spend time figuring out who was at fault and got busy figuring out how to make things better?

CHAPTER 14

Reframing

Our ability to transform anything lies in our ability to reframe it.

—Marianne Williamson, spiritual leader, activist, and author of
A Return to Love and *Healing the Soul of America*

AT FIRST glance, reframing may seem a little complicated, but bear with me. This is an amazing, life-changing technique you can use anywhere at any time to create calm in the middle of the storm, to soothe your anxiety, or to just plain feel better.

I like to think of reframing as looking at the same picture from a different angle or through a different frame. It doesn't change the event or a single detail of what happened. It simply allows you to see the facts from a different point of view. It's not asking you to pretend things are all roses and sunshine when you're in the middle of a family crisis or having a tough time financially. It's about looking at those circumstances differently. Confused?

All right, let's do a little experiment together.

Get comfortable. Now, look around at your surroundings and try to find as many things *wrong* in your environment as possible.

Is it dirty? Noisy? Smelly? What's ugly, broken, scratched? Is there clutter? Dust? Rust? Can you hear some annoying noise? Is there a dog that won't stop barking or an alarm that's been going off for hours? Is it too dark? Too bright? Too cold? Too hot?

Wow, there are a lot of things around you that could be wrong. Make a list of all the things that aren't perfect. Take your time. Be focused. Tell the truth.

1.

2.

3.

What are you thinking about your surroundings? How do you *feel* about where you are? What kind of emotions are coming up for you as you focus on the *negative*?

Write them here:

1.

2.

3.

Now take another look around the same area, but this time look for things that are *right* about the place.

Is it sunny? Clean? Is it quiet? Are you listening to some great music? Can you smell something delicious cooking or baking? Maybe there's a fresh breeze blowing through the room.

Are you comfortable? Do you have anything beautiful around you? Are there things around you that make you feel happy, calm, or joyful? Can you find a color that you love?

List three things here. Take your time. Be focused. Tell the truth.

1.

2.

3.

What are you thinking about your surroundings? How do you *feel* about where you are? What kind of emotions are coming up for you as you focus on the *positive*?

Write them here:

1.

2.

3.

As you changed your focus, did you notice a change in what you were feeling? That change in focus from negative to positive was *reframing*. The place around you hasn't changed. You haven't changed. What changed was your *focus*.

And as your focus changed from negative to positive, I bet your emotions changed, too. Now, here's some great news. Whenever you're feeling anxious, you can immediately shift the way you *feel* by shifting your *focus*.

In the same way you changed your focus from negative to positive, you can change your thinking from negative to positive.

Change my thoughts? No way, you may be thinking. *Maybe I can choose to change my focus, but there's no way I choose my thoughts. There's no way I'm choosing to think these scary thoughts. The thoughts just show up in my mind all on their own. I don't have anything to do with them. And besides, why would anyone choose to think such awful, miserably negative things on purpose?*

But if you don't choose your thoughts, who does?

The truth is, no one else can think for you. And no one else can force you to scare yourself to death with dark, terrible thoughts.

Only you can choose what you think about.

So why would a smart, capable woman like you choose to spend time making yourself sick with all these worried thoughts?

Great question.

Maybe you learned this stinking thinking as a child. Maybe your mom or dad was always looking at the dark side of things or warning you about how dangerous the world can be and it became a habit. Maybe you believe if you think those thoughts often enough, you'll somehow prevent the things you're worrying about from happening. Maybe you figure if you play enough terrifying scenarios in your head, you'll be better able to handle them when they happen in real life.

Maybe there's another reason you've been scaring yourself to death. If so, write it here:

Important: If your negative thoughts are the result of trauma and have lasted longer than six months, I recommend you don't try doing this on your own. Please seek help from a professional mental health provider. There are some amazing new techniques to help women deal with the aftereffects of trauma, especially EMDR, which has been proven to help with even the most difficult traumas.

If your negative thinking is *not* the result of trauma, let me remind you that you're choosing these negative thoughts; they're *your* thoughts, and you can change them starting right now. All you have to do is *reframe your thinking*.

Let's look at how two women used reframing to deal with their anxiety.

When Gale's doctor diagnosed her with diabetes, Gale was terrified. She worried about how she was going to follow through on her treatment plan and what lay ahead for her. But when she decided to try reframing, she began to focus on being grateful for having such a smart, competent health care provider.

She realized she was lucky to have gotten a wake-up call to change her lifestyle before it was too late. She was thankful to live in a time and place where she could get great medical care. As Gale thought differently about her diabetes, she felt more in control and ready to deal with what was ahead.

Reframing didn't change Gale's circumstances, just the way she looked at them.

When Morgan's business failed, she argued there was nothing she could possibly be grateful for. She'd failed. She'd lost every dime she'd put into her business. How could she possibly be grateful for that?

But her friend JC suggested she could be grateful for what she'd learned over the years and all the wonderful new people she'd met along the way. JC encouraged Morgan to feel proud of the courage she'd shown in tackling such a big undertaking in the first place. She reminded Morgan that she was now one of a long line of women who'd failed, then reframed that failure in a way that put them back on the road to success.

Oprah Winfrey grew up in poverty and was fired for being "unfit for TV." J. K. Rowling was a divorced, single parent living on welfare when she began writing the Harry Potter series. Her first manuscript was rejected twelve times before someone took a chance on her. (Now, that's a lot of reframing.)

The point is that these women looked at those challenges not as the end of something but as a place to begin again. And Morgan began to see she could use this setback as a way to reimagine her work and her life and then to step boldly into the future.

That's reframing.

What about you? Are you ready to think about things from a new, more positive perspective? You don't have to be glad your health is at risk or that your business failed, but there is always something you can find to be glad for. Always.

If you can't run, be glad you can walk. If you can't see, be glad you can hear. If your ship hasn't come in yet, be glad you're able to send one out.

CHAPTER 15

A Reframe of Reframing: Byron Katie's "The Work"

Do you want to meet the love of your life?
Look in the mirror.

—Byron Katie, speaker and author of *Loving What Is*
and *Your Inner Awakening*

I F YOU like the idea of reframing (see "Reframing," p. 74) but would welcome some structure to guide you, this process is for you.

Byron Katie's "The Work" is a specific set of four questions, plus what she calls "the turnaround." These questions first help you get a good look at your negative thinking and the scary stories you've been telling yourself. Then they help you to challenge that thinking and then change it.

In her own words, here's the story of how Byron Katie discovered "The Work."

I was depressed for ten years. Paranoid, agoraphobic, filled with self-loathing. Every day I wanted to die. For the last two years, I could barely leave the bedroom. Then one morning, as I lay sleeping on the floor in an attic room, a cockroach crawled over my foot. I opened my eyes, and in place of all the darkness was joy I can't describe. What I realized in that moment was that when I believed my thoughts, I suffered, and when I didn't believe my thoughts, I didn't suffer. I've come to see this is true for every human being. In that moment 'The Work' was born.

What a story of the hope and the possibilities that lie in all of us—if we're willing to risk seeing life in a new way.

As I said, Byron Katie's "The Work" is based on four simple questions and the turnaround. But those questions have the power to change the way you see yourself, your anxiety, and your world. So let's take a look at how they work.

"The Work"

Let's begin by looking at Flo, who used "The Work" to tackle her concerns about money. Flo found herself deeply in debt after being laid off and dealing with a series of medical issues.

Katie suggests you get the best results if you write down each step of the process. So Flo wrote, "I'm terrified I'm so deep in debt I'll never get out. I don't know what I'm going to do. It feels like there's no way out for me. I'm so afraid I'm going to lose my car and my condo, and that's all I have left. What will happen if I lose my health insurance?"

What's worrying you? Write it here—just the facts to start with, please.

I'm worried about

Is what you're worrying about true? Is the story you're telling yourself true?

Flo was confused by the question. Of course it was true. She had the stack of unpaid bills to prove it. She owed almost two years' worth of salary. Debt collectors were calling her night and day. Why the heck would she make up anything like that?

No question about it. The answer was "Yes, it's true."

What about your worry? Is it true?

Question Two: Is it really true? Can you absolutely know it's true?

Question two really challenges the negative stories you've been telling yourself. You may be thinking, hey, the facts are the facts. I know what's true and what's not. But wait a minute. Can you be *absolutely* sure you're still in debt, that lawsuit's still pending, or you have cancer?

What if . . . ?

When Flo started thinking about it, she admitted she wasn't *absolutely* sure she still owed all that money. She wrote, "Someone could have paid off my debt for me." "Someone could have left me a large, unexpected inheritance." "The lottery ticket in my purse could be the winning ticket." "The painting over my bed could have been painted by Monet."

As she wrote her answers, Flo was shaking her head (and maybe you are, too). *Are you kidding? You want me to swallow those ridiculous possibilities?*

82

And maybe you're thinking, "Of course I have cancer. I've seen the MRI."

But what if you're in remission? What if someone's come up with a cure?

Maybe you're arguing, "Of course that lawsuit is still pending. It's been going on for years."

But what if the person suing you has had a change of heart?

As Flo continued to argue with herself about how foolish it was to believe that the painting over her bed was anything but a nice picture of a garden, she suddenly realized how willing she'd been to believe all the terrifying stories she'd been making up about her financial woes. If she'd been ready to believe the worst, why couldn't she allow herself to believe the best? Why couldn't she tell the story differently, imagining a positive outcome, imagining the best instead of the worst?

So, how about you? What is really, really the truth about your worries?

Are those scary stories you've been telling yourself as true as you thought?

Hmmm . . .

Question Three: How do you react? What happens when you believe the thought?

This question gives a good look at the price you're paying for your negative stories. No more denial.

When Flo thought about her debt and the possibility of losing everything, she felt nauseous, hopeless, and absolutely paralyzed with fear.

How do you feel when you focus on the scary stories you've been telling yourself? Does that thought make your life better or worse? (Remember, it's just a thought/story, not the truth.)

What does that story cost you? (Be specific and honest.)

Question Four: Who would I be without that thought? What would my life look like?

Question four brought Flo a rush of relief and freedom. See if it works the same way for you.

When Flo allowed herself to think about what her life would look like without the thought that she was going to lose everything, she felt her whole body relax. And she could finally breathe again. The change was so profound, it felt almost magical.

Take a moment and think about how your life might be different if you were willing to give up or change that negative thought. Would it be better? Worse? Now describe those changes here:

How would I feel without that thought?

Are you feeling better? I hope so.

And now, the final step.

The Turnaround

The turnaround does exactly what its name suggests. It turns your thought around. It turns it inside out. It turns it on its head, just to see what happens.

When Flo took the thought "I'm so bad with money; I'll never get out of this debt" and turned it around to "I'm great with money, so I'll get out of this debt easily," her first reaction was to laugh out loud. But after a few repetitions, she was able to begin to think about ways to make that turnaround true.

All right, now you try it.

Write your worry here:

Now write your turnaround here:

Katie suggests writing three examples of a turnaround. Then ask yourself: What feels better, the original thought or the turnaround? Which feels freer? Which gives you hope? Which one is truer? What would you like to tell yourself from here on in?

By using "The Work," Flo was able to keep her focus and perspective through a few tough months, until she was able to land a great new job. She was able to find a roommate to share her condo, and by the end of the year she was well on her way to paying down that debt.

CHAPTER 16

Ask Yourself
Better Questions

*We get wise by asking questions, and even if these are not
answered, we get wise, for a well-packed question carries
its answer on its back as a snail carries its shell.*

—James Stephens, poet and author of
Irish Fairy Tales and *The Crock of Gold*

YOUR BRAIN loves to play, and one of its favorite games is
answering questions. So if you want to entertain your brain,
ask it questions. If you want to learn about life, ask questions.
If you want to deal more effectively with your anxiety and create a
new feeling of calm in your life, ask yourself *better* questions.

As Tony Robbins says, "Successful people ask better questions,
and as a result, they get better answers."

One of the things I learned early in my training as a psychotherapist was not to waste time asking my clients questions that started

with the word "why." As my former professor would say, "If people knew *why*, they wouldn't be in your office. You need to ask better questions."

She was right. I found that instead of asking "why," asking "how" or "when" or "what" was much more effective. And a more effective question *always* gets a more effective answer.

For instance, instead of asking, "*Why* am I always anxious?" ask, "*What* makes me anxious?" or "*When* am I anxious?" or "*How* could I make this better?" or "*Can* I think of steps I could take to change this situation?"

Do you see how changing a word or two can make such a dramatic difference in the quality of the answer you get? And when you change your answer, you change the emotion you feel about that answer.

Maybe changing a few words isn't going to be enough to get you a powerful answer. Maybe you need to ask a different question.

Geneen had been afraid to ride in an elevator for as long as she could remember. Just the thought of stepping into an elevator made her ask herself questions like:

"What would happen if the elevator got stuck between floors?"

"How long would it take for someone to rescue me?"

"What if I run out of air?"

"Why am I so afraid of such a stupid thing?"

"Why can't I get over this?"

"What is wrong with me?"

(Can you feel your blood pressure going up?)

What kind of answers do you think she got from these questions?

But as she began to work on her fear, Geneen began to ask herself more empowering questions like:

"What is my anxiety trying to tell me?"

"Is that useful information?"

"How could I think about this differently?"

"What thoughts could I think that would make this process easier for me?"

"Could I create an anchor or an affirmation that would make this easier?"

"Is there another tool I could use to help me feel more in control?"

"Is there someone I could ask to help me?"

Do you feel the difference between these two sets of questions?

Can you think of a question you could ask right now that might change the way you're feeling or thinking about your life or your anxiety?

How about the question "What would my life look like without anxiety?"

My favorite question of all time comes from Tony Robbins. He suggests asking, "What could I do right now to make this better?" Now, there's a great question that almost always gets a great answer.

Louise Hay recommends asking, "What thoughts can I think right now that will make me feel better?"

What if you asked yourself:

"What have I done in the past that worked?"

"Who do I know that might be able to help me through this?"

"What's one small thing I could change to make this better?"

What if you asked yourself every morning, "What wonderful thing might happen to me today?" Do you think that might change your attitude about the day ahead? Do you think you might start to look for wonderful things?

What if you asked yourself every evening before bed, "What was the best thing that happened to me today?" Do you think that question might change your focus during the day? Do you think you might start looking for wonderful things throughout the day to report on every evening?

What if you asked your children/family those questions every night? Do you think that might change their day? Their focus? Their lives?

Why not give it a try?

CHAPTER 17

The Importance of
Not Being Perfekt

I'd rather live my life knowing that I'm not perfect
than spend my whole life pretending to be.

—Will Smith, comedian, actor, rapper,
and author of *Will Smith's Rules for Success*

ARE YOU always promising yourself you're going to start a diet or an exercise program or that you are going to find a new job but somehow never get around to doing any of those things? Do you put off making important appointments? Are you great at starting projects but find yourself stalled partway through? Do you dream of taking salsa lessons or singing karaoke but feel faint at the idea of others seeing you fail at something or, worse yet, watching you make a fool of yourself in public?

Maybe, like me, you suffer from the crippling syndrome I call "perfectionitis." And we're not alone. Studies show that perfectionitis is largely a women's issue, and it impacts all areas of our lives.

We want to make sure the work we turn in is perfect. We don't go to that yoga class because we're not flexible enough (and don't even talk about putting on a pair of yoga pants with this butt, are you kidding me?). We don't speak up unless we're absolutely sure we know the answer. Sound familiar?

The need to be perfect makes us anxious, as well as causing all sorts of misery, embarrassment, and chaos.

Symptoms can include, but are not limited to: putting things off, procrastinating, not following through, feeling like you haven't done enough, haven't done it right, and everyone's going to realize you're an imposter. In short, you are not good enough!

If you are a fellow sufferer, let me share with you the good news I've found over the years.

You are *never* going to be perfect, and that's okay. Really. You are fine just the way you are. Your imperfect, funny, lovely self is just fine, without any extra accomplishments, medals, awards, degrees, bank accounts, diamonds, cars, or whatever way you've been keeping track of success. If you never earn another dollar, win another race, lose another pound, address the United Nations, or have your own TV show, you're okay. Just the way you are.

Enough Already

In her book *End the Struggle and Dance with Life*, Susan Jeffers recommends using the word "enough" as the standard to measure ourselves by. What a great idea.

What if instead of having to be perfect, you could allow yourself to be enough exactly as you are? Would you feel differently about yourself? Would you approach life differently?

What if everything you did was enough? (Not perfect, but enough.) I don't know about you, but my whole body feels lighter when I think about not having to turn myself inside out to make other people happy or to make them like me. I feel freer to try new things, to fail at things I'm trying for the first time, and to finish things even after I've realized they're not going to turn out exactly the way I'd hoped.

What if you told yourself right now that you are *always* going to be *enough*, in every circumstance, no matter what happens to you throughout the rest of your life?

What if you and everything about you was enough just the way it is right now?

Write It in Pencil

Picture yourself in the third grade. Your teacher assigns you an essay on how you spent your summer vacation. She tells you to write the essay in ink, no crossing out. No mistakes allowed, and you have only ten minutes to finish. How do you feel about the assignment?

But what if the assignment was to take your time writing that essay? What if you were told the essay didn't have to be in ink and you were given a pencil with a big, fat pink eraser you could use to correct your mistakes? Now how do you feel about the assignment? Do you feel the difference?

How often do you approach your life, your work, or your relationships as if you're writing in ink, you have a time limit, and *there can be no mistakes?*

What if you started living as if you're writing with pencil? What if your work didn't have to be perfect? What if *you* didn't have to be perfect? Would that make it easier?

What if you tossed the word "perfect" from your vocabulary?

Take a minute now and open your hands, palms up, and say, "I no longer need to be perfect. I release the need to control the outcome of what I do and what I expect. From this moment on, I allow life and/or the Divine Universe to be in charge of the future."

You are enough.

My mother's best advice to me (and she gave me a lot of great advice) was "No matter what happens to you, no matter what obstacle you face—just do your best!"

"Just do your best!"

Four simple words that can work magic in your life.

You don't have to perform miracles, cure cancer (although that would be lovely), or reinvent the wheel. All you have to do is show up, do what you can do, and stop.

Just doing your best means you get to work, sleeves rolled up to your elbows, ready to do whatever you can to make things happen. It means you work with a steady hand, focused not on the end product but on the process. It means you commit all your resources. It means you allow yourself to work fearlessly until you've done everything you can think of. Then you step back and let go of the need to control the outcome.

If things turn out well, pat yourself on the back. If they don't, remind yourself that you showed up and did your best. Stop beating yourself up. Learn from the experience and then move on.

Repeat after me, "No matter what happens, I'll just do my best."

What if I don't know what to say if they call on me in the meeting tomorrow? "I'll just do my best."

I'm terrified to buy a new car. How am I ever going to get a good price when I have to deal with the sales pitch and all that wheeling and dealing? *"I'll just do my best."*

What will I do if my child gets sick the same week I have to travel for work? *"I'll just do my best."*

What will I do if my mother's illness turns out to be serious? *"I'll just do my best."*

How do you feel when you say those words? Do they feel true? Maybe they don't right now, but what if they were true? Can you imagine that? What would your life look like? What would your anxiety feel like? Why not find out?

CHAPTER 18

Let Go

Some people believe holding on and hanging in there are signs of great strength. However, there are times when it takes much more strength to know when to let go and then to do it.

—Ann Landers, advice columnist and author of
Wake Up and Smell the Coffee!

WHAT IF you've tried everything you can think of to change your negative thinking and nothing's worked? What if you've asked questions, tried affirmations, reframed, regrouped, and ate the last piece of chocolate cake, and you're still feeling lousy? What then?

Well, how about resigning as Ms. Grand Pooh-bah of the Universe, relaxing a little, and just letting go of your burdens, fears, and worries for a while?

What if you released all your "what ifs," the "musts," the "shoulds," and the "have tos"? How would it feel to be able to stop rowing upstream and let the current gently carry you downstream for a time?

Maybe you're arguing that you can't possibly put down all the responsibilities you're carrying. You have children. You have parents. People need you. You're in charge. You're necessary. The world won't turn without you. And besides, you can't just let go of those worried thoughts. They're a part of you. They're necessary to keep you productive, functioning, and safe. There's no way you can just let go of them or anything else.

But what if you could?

Here are three methods that can help you do just that.

The Sedona Method

This simple technique suggests you ask yourself a series of easy questions that allow you to release difficult or unwanted emotions.

So, how does the method work? Let's take a look at how Lori used the Sedona Method in her life.

Step One: Focus on any issue you would like to feel better about. Lori worried constantly that people would notice the skin condition affecting her back and shoulders. She wore long sleeves year-round and dreaded the warm weather because she had to make all sorts of excuses for not wearing sundresses, halter tops, or bathing suits. She knew worry made her condition worse, but she couldn't help it. When Lori decided to try the Sedona Method, her first step was to focus on her anxiety about that skin condition.

Step Two: Ask yourself *one* of these three questions. Remember, there are no wrong answers here. Both "yes" and "no" are acceptable.

1. Could I let this feeling go?

2. Could I allow this feeling to be here?

3. Could I welcome this feeling?

Lori asked herself if she could let go of her worry about her skin condition and immediately answered with a loud "No way." She certainly couldn't welcome the feeling and didn't want it to be a part of her life.

Step Three: Once you've answered your question from step two, ask yourself again, "Could I let this feeling go?" If the answer is yes, go on to step four. If the answer is no, ask yourself, "Would I rather have this feeling, or would I rather be free?"

No matter what you answer, go on to step four.

As Lori thought about how miserable all that worry was making her, she began to wonder what life would be like if she could be free of it. She imagined herself wearing a sundress on a warm summer afternoon and enjoying the warmth of the sun on her shoulders. And she wondered what it would be like to let go of the feelings that had been running her life.

Step Four: Ask yourself, "When?" If your answer isn't "now," ask again, reminding yourself that you're in charge of this process and can let go anytime you choose. If you're still feeling stuck and unwilling to let go, move on to step five.

Lori decided to take a chance and release her worries right then and there.

Step Five: Repeat steps one through four as necessary until you're free of any of those unwanted feelings you started with in step one. It took Lori a while to let go of those long-held worries. But once she started to release those feelings, she found she was able to relax around other people, and over time her skin condition improved.

The Sedona Method looks and sounds simple, but don't let that simplicity fool you. This method works for lots of people. Why not give it a try?

The Pink Bubble Technique

The first time I came across the idea of "letting go" was in Shakti Gawain's book *Creative Visualization*. In it, Shakti described an amazing technique called the "Pink Bubble Technique." This visualization involves mentally enclosing your goals and wishes in a pink bubble and releasing them into the universe in order to attract energy for manifestation of those goals.

I loved the idea but decided to use her pink bubble in a different way. Instead of mentally sending my fondest wishes into the atmosphere, I used the technique to get rid of the negative thoughts that were running my life.

Of course, you can use this technique in whatever way works best for you. Try them both if you like. Switch them up. Add your own special touches to make them work for *you*.

Let Your Worries Go

Begin by relaxing fully. Now focus on some thought or emotion you no longer want in your life. Imagine that thought or emotion encircled in a clear pink bubble or balloon. Picture yourself walking along the beach or any place that feels peaceful to you. You're holding the string to that balloon of negativity that floats over your head. As you walk along the beach, watch the water, enjoy the day, and smell the salt in the air until you feel it's exactly the right moment to let go of the string.

When you're ready, open your hand. The instant the string leaves your hand, notice the feeling of having that weight lifted off your shoulders. Enjoy the freedom that comes from letting go of worries, fears, and doubts.

As always, how you use this technique is completely up to you. If you don't want to imagine a walk on the beach, you can imagine yourself on top of a building in New York or on a mountain in Nepal. If you don't want to use a pink bubble, use an orange or green one.

You can use the pink bubble every morning to send out your wishes for the day and at night to release the day's troubles. Please do what's right for you. Let go of having to do things the "right" way.

Worry About It Tomorrow

Probably the most famous way of letting go of your worries comes from *Gone with the Wind*. Remember Scarlett O'Hara's famous speech about putting off her worry until later? She says, "I can't think about this now. I'll go crazy if I do. I'll think about it tomorrow."

What do you think would happen if you refused to allow yourself to worry today about anything at all? What if you put off thinking about those concerns until tomorrow? And what if you did the same thing tomorrow? The way I see it, using this technique will allow you to live a worry-free life one day at a time.

CHAPTER 19

Take Action

*Twenty years from now you will be more disappointed
by the things you didn't do than the ones you did. So throw
off the bowlines, sail away from the safe harbor. Catch the
trade winds in your sails. Explore. Dream. Discover.*

—Mark Twain, humorist and author of
The Adventures of Huckleberry Finn and *The Adventures of Tom Sawyer*

TAKE A minute and write down the three biggest worries in
your life right now.

1.

2.

3.

Now let's take those worries and get to work creating a plan to deal with them in a way that works for you.

Turning Your Worries into an Action Plan

Step One: Pick the one worry that weighs you down the most.

Now write down everything you know about it. Be specific. Name names. Write the who, what, where, when, how, and why of your anxiety. Really take a hard look about what's bothering you and put it all down on paper.

For instance, Janice was concerned about her relationship with her sister, Kate. They'd never been close, but after the death of their mother, they'd fought over who was going to inherit their mother's ring, her two gold bracelets, and her diamond necklace.

Step Two: Write down all the possible solutions to your problem. Start with the obvious. Then move on to the "not so obvious." Really think outside the box here. Be silly, have fun, suspend reason, and let loose. How would your best friend solve this problem? Mother Teresa? The Queen of England? Taylor Swift? What if you could put a call in to Rosa Parks or Marie Curie and get their input? What might they tell you?

After some thought, Janice wrote:

1. Mother Teresa would forgive Kate, apologize, and let Kate have the necklace.
2. Taylor Swift would write a song about what a jerk Kate was and make a million dollars in the process.
3. The Queen of England would order Kate to return both bracelets, then sentence her to serve time in the Tower of London.
4. Marie Curie would examine the facts from all sides and find a logical solution.
5. Rosa Parks would look for an equitable solution and take bold action to make sure justice was served.

Now it's your turn. Write down as many ideas as you can. Don't judge, just write. (You can laugh if you like.) How many ideas do you have? Could you think of just two more? Go ahead.

Like Janice, feel free to push beyond the limits of what you know to what might be possible. Some of the world's best ideas have come from crazy thinking. And by challenging yourself this way, you may come up with an amazing solution that you never would have considered otherwise. Maybe you could combine two of your ideas into the perfect solution. Give it a try.

Step Three: All right, now let's look at the list of solutions you've created. Some will make sense, some will not. Some will be possible, some will not. That's fine.

The next step is to rule out the solutions you're sure will never work.

Janice dismissed the idea of the best-selling song and sentencing Kate to the Tower of London.

Now, go down that list, draw a line through the absolute losers, and circle the solutions that make the most sense to you. I recommend you look for the ideas that seem the most fun, feel the most inspiring or the most practical, or simply resonate with you.

If you have more than three ideas, the next step is to choose the top three and put a check mark beside them. Once you have narrowed your choice down to three possible answers, you're going to rank them in order (1 being most likely to 3 being least likely).

Write them here:

1.

2.

3.

Your number one choice is where you're going to start. If you find your first option doesn't work, you'll have a backup plan in your second and third choices.

1. After reviewing the facts carefully, Janice came up with what felt like an equitable solution and a plan to approach Kate with that solution.
2. If that didn't work, Janice decided she would return the disputed necklace to her sister and wait to see her response.
3. If neither of those ideas worked, Janice decided she would be all right with that, too, knowing she had done the best she could.

Step Four: Take action. Hopefully you've created an action plan that's so inspiring or exciting that you can't wait to take action. But if you're already talking yourself into not following through, why not start by taking just one small action toward your goal? Stop. Give yourself a pat on the back. Then, when you're ready, take another step. (See "Just Do One Small Thing," p. 122.)

Janice called Kate and they worked together to create a plan for dividing the jewelry that satisfied them both. They met briefly to exchange the jewelry.

Step Five: Once you've taken action, take a few minutes to evaluate how effective it was. Did it work the way you'd planned? If not, how could you have done it differently? Are you willing to make a few changes in your approach and try again? Or do you think it would be more effective to try a whole new approach? If so, go back to your list, pick your second solution, and put it into action.

Although their relationship wasn't healed overnight, Janice felt much better about her relationship with her sister and hoped things would continue to improve.

Step Six: Repeat this process until the problem lessens or disappears.

CHAPTER 20

Face Your Fears

*You gain strength, courage, and confidence by every
experience in which you really stop to look fear in the face.
You must do the thing you think you cannot do.*

—Eleanor Roosevelt, diplomat, activist,
and former first lady of the United States

S O YOU read the title of this chapter and you're arguing, "Are
you nuts? Do you really think I'm going to be able to stand
up to _____(write the thing you fear most
on this planet)? If I could do that, I wouldn't be reading this book.
I'd be out living a great, anxiety-free life. Just that title makes my
palms sweat."

I felt the same way, until I read a great book called *Feel the Fear
and Do It Anyway*. (If you haven't read *Feel the Fear*, or any of Susan
Jeffers's books, I highly recommend them.)

Jeffers lets us know right up front that every time you tackle
something new, you're going to be afraid. And the only way to

conquer that fear is to do the thing that you fear most.

Maybe that's not what you were hoping to hear, but it's the truth. We're all afraid. But if you look around, you'll see that some women let their fear hold them back, while other women step boldly into the unknown. The question is, which one will you choose to be?

As Les Brown, the incredible motivational speaker, says, none of us can hide from life. None of us can sit on the bleachers of life, forever, watching everyone else dance. No matter how scared we are, no matter how we hide, sooner or later life is going to drag us out onto the dance floor, so we'd better learn some steps.

The reality is both the women on the bleachers and the women who take the risk and dance anyway feel fear. But the women who risk and dance anyway get to have the fun and excitement of dancing and being a part of things, while the women sitting on the bleachers may be left with nothing but regrets at missing yet another chapter of their life. *I should have made that call. I wish I wasn't so afraid to fly; I'm missing so much. I wish I'd taken that risk. I should have . . . I'm ashamed I didn't . . .*

So how do you find the courage to take that first step? Let's look at the anatomy of fear.

Jeffers's Three Levels of Fear

Level One

This level includes our external fears, the scary things that happen *outside* us and keep us awake at night. These external fears can be broken into two types. The first are all those things that happen *to* us: for instance, aging, natural disasters, war, death, et cetera. These are things we can't do anything about.

The other type of external fears are the ones that *require us to take action*: for instance, facing your boss, ending or beginning a relationship, giving a speech, flying, et cetera.

As you read over these lists, I bet you're coming up with your own list of external fears.

Write them here:

1.

2.

3.

Level Two

The second level includes those fears you create *inside* you. These are the learned fears that may be running your life without you even being aware of it. They include: fear of rejection, of failure, of being alone, of being abandoned, et cetera.

Again, you're probably coming up with a list of those internal fears that play on a loop in your mind and keep you stuck and afraid.

Write them here:

1.

2.

3.

Level Three

This level goes the deepest and in the end is the only fear that matters. You may be surprised to learn there's just one fear listed here, but it is the single fear that creates and feeds all the fears listed above. Honestly, this is the secret menace that keeps us all prisoners to all those other fears.

Are you ready to lift the curtain and look directly into the face of what you are afraid of? Here we go.

"I can't handle it!"

That's it. That one fear is the source of all our other fears. If we send this fear packing, the others will go with it.

Not convinced yet? Stick with me as we look at this more closely. Go back to the lists you've created above and, as Jeffers recommends, put the phrase "I'm afraid . . ." in front of each one of your fears.

Now read each one aloud, and as you say each phrase, see what kind of feelings come up for you.

"I'm afraid I won't be able to handle this move."

"I'm afraid I won't be able to handle this major exam."

"I'm afraid I will never be able to leave my house again."

How are you feeling? Afraid? Worried?

But what if you changed both the phrase and the thought that you're not capable of handling your life? What if you starting telling yourself you are capable of taking care of yourself and anything that happens to you? What if you decided to start trusting yourself? So let's change the phrase "I'm afraid I can't handle" to "I trust I *can* handle . . ."

"I trust I can handle this move."

"I trust I can handle this major exam."

"I trust I will be able to leave my house again."

Do you feel a shift in your thinking? I know I did.

I Am Not Alone

As I've played with this concept over the years, I've found I could increase my sense of peace and calm a hundredfold by acknowledging that I'm not traveling this road alone. Instead of just saying, "I can handle anything that happens to me," I broaden this phrase to include the concept of God (spirit companion, guide, angel, ancestor, saint, life force, or any other spiritual concept that appeals to you). "I, and the Divine within me, can handle anything that happens to me."

When I include this divine traveling companion in this phrase, it takes on a new depth and power in my life.

That really works for me. It may not work at all for you, and that's fine, too. In fact, you may come up with your own vision of how to use this concept that works perfectly for you and looks completely different. Great. There's no right or wrong way of doing this work; there's just your way of facing and healing your fear.

In the end, fear is a part of life and something we're all going to have to deal with. So why not put on a pair of dancing shoes, try out a few new steps, and get ready to hit the dance floor.

CHAPTER 21

DIY Affirmations

*When I talk about affirmations, I mean consciously
choosing words that will either help eliminate something
from your life or help create something new in your life.*

—Louise Hay, motivational speaker and author of
You Can Heal Your Life and *The Power Is Within You*

FIRST RAN across the idea of using affirmations in Louise Hay's book *You Can Heal Your Life*. I loved the idea that I could change my life by changing the way I thought and I could change the way I thought by affirming the positive.

I immediately started playing with affirmations and have been using them ever since.

So what's an affirmation?

An affirmation is a confident statement. A *good* affirmation is always positive. It's always stated in the first person, as if you already have the positive result you're asking for. The more specific and personal you can make that statement, the better. The more uplifting and joyful you can make those details, the better.

For instance:

"I wish I could afford a new coat this year" becomes "I love wearing my new warm cashmere coat to work every morning." Do you *feel* the difference?

"I'll never find a perfect partner" becomes "I so enjoy spending time with this wonderful person who makes my heart sing every time I'm with him/her."

Here's the most important thing of all about affirmations. *You don't have to believe what you're affirming.* You just have to be willing to repeat it and be open to the idea that through repetition you're going to change what you believe. And when you change what you believe, you can change your life.

While any affirmation that resonates with you can work, I've found the most effective affirmations are the ones you create yourself. So let's take a few minutes to build a list of affirmations that work for you.

First I'm going to ask you to write down some of your most negative thoughts. Let me get you started with some of the comments women have shared with me over the years.

"I'm not good enough."

"I hate my body."

"I'll never be able to afford that."

"I don't deserve a raise."

"I can't do that."

"Women can't do that."

Now spend some time focusing on those dark, debilitating thoughts you don't share with anyone else. Write them in any order you like, and don't be shy or hold back.

Put your thoughts here:

1.

2.

3.

Once you're done, let's sit together a moment while you experience some of the feelings that come up for you as you focus on these negative thoughts. If you like, you can write those feelings here, naming them as specifically as you can. Are you angry? Sad? Lonely? Afraid? Depressed? Anxious?

Put all those difficult emotions on the table once and for all.

Write your feelings here in as much detail as you can:

1.

2.

3.

Now get ready to replace those negative thoughts and feelings with some positive, uplifting affirmations.

Pick the worst thought you were able to come up with. For instance:

> Olivia hated herself for smoking and was ashamed she couldn't seem to quit. When asked to write her most negative thoughts about it, Olivia wrote, "I hate myself for not being able to give up this disgusting habit. I hate having to go outside at work to smoke. I hate how friends and family look at me when I light up. I hate myself for being such a failure."

Write your most miserable, negative thought here:

Olivia wrote, "I feel hopeless, ashamed, and angry at myself. I hate myself for being so weak and spineless."

Are you feeling as miserable as I am?

All right—let's make a change.

Let's focus on the exact opposite of those lousy thoughts.

For instance, Olivia wrote, "It feels wonderful to be smoke-free. I am so proud of my accomplishment. People around me are proud as well. I am able to handle what life brings my way. I am proud of myself."

Write the opposites of those lousy thoughts here:

1.

2.

3.

Now you have several new affirmations you can use. You can use one or all of them. It's up to you.

Once you've created the affirmation that feels just right for you, make it your screen saver. Write it on a Post-it Note and tape it up on the bathroom mirror, where you'll see it every day.

Read it aloud as often as you can. Repeat it to yourself when you're in traffic or showering. The more you repeat the statement, the more it becomes a part of you.

Olivia used affirmations as an important part of her successful plan to quit smoking, and she continues to use them in other aspects of her life.

Like Olivia, you can create an affirmation for every negative thought you have and then use them until they become true in your life.

Affirmations are like jumping jacks or sit-ups. The more you do them, the stronger you get. Start now to strengthen your thinking and your emotional health. You're worth it.

CHAPTER 22

Accentuate the Positive

Everyone is a genius. But if you judge a fish on its ability to climb a tree, it will live its whole life believing it is stupid.

—Albert Einstein

The Confidence Gap

Over the last few years, women have come a long way in the workplace. But we still have a way to go. According to "The Confidence Gap" by Katty Kay and Claire Shipman, published in the *Atlantic*, "Men around us have continued to get promoted faster and be paid more." And today women hold fewer than 19 percent of the board seats on Fortune 1000 companies. What's holding us back?

There are certainly still institutional barriers in place. And we're still more likely to take time off to care for children and aging parents. But the real reason we haven't been able to shatter that glass ceiling is something called the "confidence gap."

Research shows that many of us are anxious about being good enough. We tell ourselves we're not smart enough. We tell ourselves our work has to be perfect before we turn it in. No misspelled words or missing commas for us. (See "The Importance of Not Being Perfekt," p. 89.) When women fail at something, they blame themselves. When men fail, they blame the economy, the boss, and everything else in the universe but themselves.

We don't speak up in meetings unless we're sure we have the right answer. We don't ask for raises.

Even successful women report feeling like imposters and that they don't deserve their success.

Yikes!

So how do we get past the worry that we're not good enough? By focusing on our strengths, our talents, and our skills.

What Do You Do Well?

What do you do well?

Are you stumped by the question?

I bet if I asked you to list your failures, shortcomings, and weaknesses, you'd have no trouble coming up with a long list of things you don't like about yourself. You may be thinking you could write a book about your mistakes, your screwups, and all the ways you don't measure up, especially that stupid thing you did that everyone's still talking about.

As you think those thoughts, how are you feeling? Are you inspired to take action, or are you beating yourself up again for not being perfect?

All right, put those negative thoughts aside and let's take a look at your successes, triumphs, and strengths. How many can you come up with?

If you're like most women, you may be having trouble listing more than one or two positives about yourself, because you haven't done much thinking about what makes you so special. That's okay. This is a great time to start telling your story a different way.

Take a minute and read this list of wonderful qualities. Circle the ones that apply to you. Don't be modest. If the word applies even a little, circle it. Even the smallest positive strength can be used to bring a sense of calm to your life.

List of Positive Aspects

attractive	fair	judicious
authentic	faithful	kind
aware	far-sighted	knowledgeable
balanced	firm	leader
bold	flexible	logical
brave	focused	loving
brilliant	forthright	purposeful
broad-minded	freewheeling	quiet
business-like	friendly	rational
calm	frugal	realistic
candid	funny	reflective
capable	generous	relaxed
charming	gentle	reliable
cheerful	genuine	resilient
clear	good-natured	resourceful
clever	graceful	respectful
compassionate	gracious	responsible
competent	grateful	responsive
confident	happy	risk-taker
congenial	hardworking	romantic
connected	helpful	self-confident
conscientious	honest	self-controlled
constant	honorable	self-reliant
daring	imaginative	sensitive
decisive	independent	sensual
dedicated	innovative	serious
elegant	inquisitive	thoughtful
emotional	insightful	tidy
empathic	intelligent	unassuming
energetic	intentional	understanding
enthusiastic	intuitive	warmhearted
entrepreneurial	involved	willing
expressive	joyful	

Once you've circled all the items that apply to you, write them here:

1.

2.

3.

4.

5.

6.

7.

8.

Now let's go a little deeper.
What are you good at?

1. Do you have a special talent?

2. What achievement makes you proudest?

3. What qualities have you used in the past to help you successfully cope with your anxiety?

4. What's the nicest compliment you've ever received?

5. What have friends and family told you about your special gifts?

6. What have teachers, bosses, and other professionals told you about your strengths?

7. What qualities and gifts would you like to be remembered for?

8. What great qualities would you mention first on your résumé?

9. Can you think of anything to add to your list? Please list those other gifts here:

As you read your list of your successes, strengths, and talents, how do you feel? Better? Stronger? Less anxious?

What if you built your future successes from the solid foundation of your past successes and your personal strengths? How would you feel going forward?

Let's begin by focusing on the three qualities you know for sure you can rely on in good times and in bad. Remember, there are no right or wrong answers here, just the answers that best describe you.

List your three positive aspects here:

1.

2.

3.

Now, how are we going to put those three amazing strengths to work in your life?

Here's an example of how Alice used her personal strengths to face the anxiety of finding a new job.

When Alice lost her job, she'd worried she wouldn't be able to find work again. The job market was tough at best. But she decided to identify her strengths and use them to help in her job search.

After reading over the list of positive aspects, she came up with twelve positive qualities she felt defined her. Then she identified the three she believed were her strongest—persistence, kindness, and creativity.

After some thought, Alice decided she could depend on her persistence to help her stick with it even in the face of disappointment or rejection. She wouldn't quit because she had a tough day. She could count on herself to see things through.

She realized she could rely on her kindness to nurture herself through the process of sending out résumés, interviewing, and networking. That sense of being loved and cared for helped her ease her anxious feelings and helped her to remain positive in the face of disappointment.

And she could depend on her creativity to think outside the box about possible jobs. She thought about changing careers, debated going back to school to learn some new skills, and considered moving.

She worked on creating a standout résumé and came up with a unique way to contact the person doing the hiring. In the end she decided to volunteer at a company that later hired her as a full-time employee.

Now, what about you?

What's making you anxious? Write it here:

How could you use the first of those three positive traits to help you deal with that worry?

How could you use the second of those three positive traits to help you?

How could use the third of those three positive traits to help you?

So there you have it. Instead of focusing on your weaknesses and failures, you've now identified at least three powerful, positive qualities that can help you get through your most difficult days with ease, grace, and love.

As you begin to see how strong, talented, and capable you really are, you won't be so afraid to speak up for yourself or trust that you'll be able to meet the unknown challenges at work and at home with a quiet, confident sense of calm and purpose.

CHAPTER 23

Just Do One Small Thing: The Art of Kaizen

Courage is one step ahead of fear.

—Coleman Young, activist, politician, and former mayor of Detroit

Kaizen:
1. A business philosophy or system that is based on making
positive changes on a regular basis, as to improve productivity.
2. An approach to one's personal or social life that
focuses on continuous improvement.
Origin: Japanese: literally, "continuous improvement"

—Taken from dictionary.reference.com

PSST. I have a secret. Come a little closer and I'll tell you how to tiptoe past the dragon of fear that stands guard in your brain and keeps you from getting what you want in life. You know the one I mean, that green, scaly creature that paces back and forth in your brain or lies coiled and waiting in your amygdala (see "The Anxious Brain," p. 3) just to roar to life at your first hint of a thought of danger or fear. Feel free to picture the monster/dragon any way that feels right to you. After all, you know it best.

You can give it a name if you'd like or draw a picture of it here:

The more you get to know the monster, the better you'll be at taming it.

Now, are you ready to know the secret to succeeding at almost anything in life?

Here it is: *Take small steps.*

That's how you slip past that dragon of fear in your brain. That's how you get past the anxiety that's been running your life. Take the smallest step possible toward your goal, celebrate that tiny success, and then take the next step. It's that simple.

When your steps are small, there's almost no danger of failure. And when there's no fear of failure, there's no anxiety to waken the dragon. What could be easier? What could be more freeing?

That's kaizen—*taking small steps toward a better life.*

The philosophy of kaizen has been used in industry for years to help companies deal with change and create better products.

Here's a look at how Kristie put kaizen to work for her.

When Kristie's beautiful baby girl, Crystal, was eight weeks old, Kristie went back to work. With long days at work and even longer sleepless nights, Kristie felt like she was on the clock twenty-four hours a day. She was exhausted, anxious, and overwhelmed.

Everyone told her she looked awful and should take time for herself. The problem was she had no idea how she was supposed to find time in her schedule to get to the gym, have a mani/pedi, or meditate when there were days she didn't have time to take a shower. And how was she supposed to eat better when she was eating take-out at least six nights a week?

Kristie was at her wit's end when she heard about kaizen from a coworker. Although the coworker was suggesting they use it at work, Kristie loved the idea of using it to practice self-care at home.

She couldn't get to the gym, but she could do a push-up while she waited for the formula to heat or she could take a two-minute walk after lunch. She could meditate for a minute between clients, and she could make some healthier choices at the drive-through window.

Not only did making these small changes help Kristie feel better physically, but they also helped her feel like she was more in control of her time and her life. And she knew it helped make her a better parent to Crystal.

Your Turn

Let's imagine you have a big, wonderful, exciting goal you want to achieve. Something you've been dreaming of for a while, but anxiety has always kept you from going after it.

Take a moment and think about what you've been too afraid to tackle. Maybe it's losing weight, starting an exercise plan, finding a partner, getting a job, or healing your anxiety. Make sure this is a goal that resonates with you.

Write that goal here:

Now take a minute and think about that goal. If you're already feeling panicked and are busy telling yourself that the goal isn't possible, I want you to take a deep breath. Relax and know you now have a wonderful new way to slip past that waiting dragon, together.

In his book *One Small Step Can Change Your Life*, Robert Maurer, PhD, lays out a series of small steps you can take to break that big, scary goal into manageable sections.

Ask smaller questions. Kristie found that instead of asking herself, "How am I ever going to get my prepregnancy body back?" asking, "What's one small thing I could do right now to feel better?" helped her feel less helpless and more like taking action.

If you want to lose weight, instead of asking, "How am I going to lose fifty pounds?" (see "Ask Yourself Better Questions," p. 86), ask, "What is the smallest possible step I could take today to move toward this goal?"

If your dragon so much as opens an eye, the step is too big. Go smaller. Maybe you're not ready to eat more vegetables, but could you look up a vegetable recipe or two? Maybe you're not ready to drink more water, but could you think about buying a water bottle to carry with you? (See "Heal with Water," p. 251.)

Whether you want to write a symphony, lower your blood sugar, or create a calm-centered life, repeatedly asking small, positive questions will get you small, useful answers.

Take small actions. Don't be afraid that the step you're taking is too small; that's just not possible. The smaller the steps you take, the better.

If you want to start your own company, you don't have to create the logo, get a loan, and start hiring employees this afternoon. But could you glance at a few websites of people/companies doing something similar? Could you doodle a few ideas on a napkin at lunch? Too scary? Too big?

Fine, make it smaller. Just turn on the computer today. Just find a blank napkin. Tomorrow you'll be able to take the next small step to success, because of the small step you've taken today. I think of this process as a way to build your wall of success brick by tiny brick. No matter how small the brick, it's still another step in building that wall and accomplishing your goal.

Taking the smallest possible action allows you to creep past that dragon of fear without waking it.

So step out fearlessly.

The moment you feel stuck or resistant, the answer is always: *Think smaller.* Make your questions, your thinking, and your actions smaller and go get the life you've been waiting to have.

Solve problems when they're small. Ahh, this is such a good one. My grandmother (and maybe yours, too) used to say, "A stitch in time saves nine." That's what we're talking about here.

Solve the problem when it's just a tiny crack in your ceiling, not when the plaster is falling into your morning coffee. Sew that button back on before you lose it. Go to the dentist for that toothache.

All right, solving problems is easy to do for the really obvious things, but what about the disaster that seems to come from nowhere without warning?

Let me suggest there may have been some warning signs that you've missed along the way. There are lights in my car that come on when I need gas or air in my tires or when the engine is in serious trouble. Wouldn't it be great if life came with the same kind of warning system?

Well, it does, sort of. The trouble is that some of the clues are subtle, and we can overlook them in the busyness of daily life. So the first step here is to pay attention to that inner voice that whispers to you that something's not working. We all have that inner sense that tells us when we get off track, but some of us are more accustomed to listening to and trusting its guidance than others.

Have you ever had a sense that something was wrong? Or something was exactly right? How did you know? Did it show up in your body, or did you feel it emotionally?

No matter how your guidance shows up for you, that feeling is your inner guidance system. And getting in touch with that system can give you some incredibly important information about keeping you and your life on track in the face of life's obstacles.

So what's one small way you could listen to that inner guidance today? How would things change for you if you trusted that inner voice?

If you really want to create a calm center in your life, fixing the small stuff when it's still small can give you a sense of confidence that comes from knowing you're doing everything you can to take care of yourself.

If you're ready to tiptoe past the scaly green dragon of anxiety, go small.

CHAPTER 24

Gratitude

Give thanks for unknown blessings on their way.

—Native American saying

W HEN JOAN'S eight-year-old son, Andrew, was diagnosed with a severe learning disability, she was terrified. She felt alone, afraid, and anxious. She lay awake nights wondering what kind of treatment he would need, how she was going to be able to pay for it, and what the future held for her son.

She dreaded the appointments with professionals, and she hated the long drive to and from those appointments with her son. Then, one afternoon, as they were heading home from a particularly discouraging appointment, her son said, "Mom, we're so lucky."

"Why are we lucky?" Joan asked, thinking the exact opposite was true.

"Lots of reasons," Andrew said. "We have such a good car. It's always warm when we go places, and when we're in the car we get to talk to each other, just the two of us."

"Really?" Joan was shocked to hear that her son didn't see the long drives as an annoyance but as a chance to spend time together. And it certainly hadn't occurred to her to be grateful for her car. But when she thought about it, she realized Andrew was right. They were lucky to have a good car, and it was a gift to be able to spend time with her son.

"You're right," she said. And as she spoke, she realized she was no longer worrying about what was ahead. She was appreciating what she had in the present. Her shoulders relaxed and she smiled at her son.

"And we're lucky because we get to have pizza tonight," Andrew continued.

Joan nodded and said back to him playfully, "And we're lucky because it isn't raining today."

And they continued to find reasons why they were lucky all the way home. They made it a game and played it in the car, in waiting rooms, and every night at bedtime.

Joan began taking time every day to find lucky things all through the day to share with Andrew. And as she focused more on what she was grateful for, she was able to see the support and love around her that she could count on in the days ahead and she felt far less anxious.

And Joan's not alone. Studies have found that grateful women report feeling better physically and emotionally. They tend to sleep better and to have better self-esteem.

How does gratitude work? Alex Korb, PhD, explains in his blog that our brains can't focus on negative and positive thoughts at the same time. (Go ahead, give it a try. Think of both a dancing blue elephant and your tax bill. See, it's just not possible.) So, when you're concentrating on the great things in your life, your brain can't dwell on those scary, anxious thoughts. What could be better than that?

Take a minute and think of three things you're grateful for right now.

If you can't think of anything, why not start with your wonderful body. Are you grateful for your sight? Hearing? Breathing? Walking?

Now, take a step outside yourself and look around at your immediate environment.

What people, places, or things are you grateful for? Once you've listed them, move beyond your environment to the broader world. What are you grateful for in your community? Your city/town? Your country? Your planet? Your universe?

Write them here:

Ways to Practice Gratitude

One way to practice gratitude is to keep a gratitude journal. Recording what you're grateful for every day keeps your focus on things in the present. It also gives you a record of the wonderful things you already have in your life that you'll be able to revisit on darker days.

You can use a few words to describe what you're grateful for, or you can write paragraphs of detailed description. You can even draw or cut out pictures of those gratitudes. Do what works best for you.

Do you think you could come up with two or three new gratitudes every day? Don't worry if you can't. Some things are so amazing that they're worth mentioning over and over (chocolate and Sunday brunch come to mind). Remember, you're the boss here—you choose.

Consider keeping a gratitude jar, which works along the lines of a worry box (see "The Worry Box," p. 268). I love the idea of writing two or three gratitudes a day on small slips of paper and tossing them into a large, clear jar so you can watch the pile grow.

What a wonderful resource to have on hand when times are tough. You can reach in and pull out as many gratitudes as you need to remind you of all the good things you've already experienced along the way.

Don't be shy about sharing your gratitude with others. Write a thank-you note to someone who helped you through a tough time. Leave a great review online. Call a family member or a friend and tell them what they mean to you and how important they are in your life. When you share your gratitude with others, it will grow and flourish in your own life as well.

CHAPTER 25

Faith

Faith is the bird that feels the light when the dawn is still dark.

—Rabindranath Tagore, Nobel Prize–winning poet, musician, artist, and author of *The Home and the World*

MY FIRST reaction to the news I had breast cancer (after the shock and fear wore off) was *This is not fair!* I was taking great care of myself physically. I was running, eating well, getting plenty of rest. I had yearly physicals. I had followed all the rules and gotten cancer anyway. This was *not* supposed to happen!

In those early months after the diagnosis, the first surgery, and the beginning of chemo, I alternated between fear, sorrow, exhaustion, and anger at this unfair twist of fate. I felt singled out for what felt like an undeserved punishment, and I felt very much alone.

Then, one dark night, I was lying awake, wondering how I was ever going to get through the next day, when I suddenly felt the presence of the Divine. There were no trumpets, no bright lights, no choirs of angels, just a quiet sense of a comforting presence in me and around me. It allowed me to finally fall into a deep, healing sleep. The next morning, I was not convinced that presence had been anything but a dream, because until that night, faith had little meaning for me and no place in my life.

That morning I realized what I'd been doing wasn't working anymore. I was too tired, too broken to go on alone. So I challenged God to prove his presence, and I waited . . .

That afternoon I was standing on an athletic field watching a soccer game. When I looked up, I saw one small, wispy cloud overhead in the otherwise blue sky. And in the middle of that cloud was a small, glorious rainbow. No joke.

I stared for a moment, looked away, then looked back. It was still there.

It was clear and beautiful and completely unexplainable scientifically. That was the moment I felt my life shift.

Over the next few weeks I read, asked questions, and wrestled with my long-held secular view of the world, as this new road of faith beckoned. In the end, I realized faith is a *choice*. You don't have to be born into a faith. You don't have to take anyone else's word for what you believe, because no one else knows any more than you do about the mysteries of this world and beyond. *What you believe is your choice.*

I could choose to continue battling through life on my own, or I could accept and welcome the presence of the Divine. I chose faith. I continue to choose faith and the sense of calm and love that comes from the realization that I am never alone.

As Wayne Dyer says, "If you knew who walks beside you on the way you have chosen, fear would be impossible."

And for me, belief has brought a sense of ease and joy into my life that nothing else has ever matched.

Ways to Connect with Your Spirit

Meditation is a great way to make that connection with the spirit within (see "Meditate," p. 146). I find visualization works well for me, but I suggest you try more than one technique to find the one that works best for you.

Be open to possibilities. I certainly didn't expect to see a rainbow in a blue sky, and I've found that spirit often shows up in surprising ways and in unexpected places. So let go of your expectations and be ready to be astonished at the way spirit reveals itself in your life.

Go for a nature walk. Being outside offers endless opportunities for God to show up. Be patient. Sometimes spirit doesn't respond immediately. Sometimes the answer takes days or even weeks—so hang in there. I promise, the answer is on its way.

I've shared my story here, but maybe you come from a different place faith-wise. Maybe you're already living a life based on the foundation of faith. Maybe your faith is in yourself, in science, or in the divine order of the universe. Maybe faith is something you used to have in your life and might want back. Maybe you're living a wonderful life without any interest in thinking or talking about any of this faith thing.

As I said, what you believe or don't believe is always your choice. There are no right or wrong answers, just the answers that work for *you*.

How to Be Fully Alive in This Hour (FAITH)

When I was going through six months of chemo for breast cancer, I struggled with exhaustion and an anxiety so intense I had trouble getting out of bed every morning. Just when I started to think I wasn't going to be able to go on one more day, I heard Scott O'Grady speak.

As you may or may not remember, Captain Scott O'Grady was an air force fighter pilot whose F-16C was shot down over Bosnia in June 1995. I remember hearing him describe how he'd survived behind enemy lines before being rescued. As he talked about the thought-tool he'd used to keep himself focused, alert, and alive, I realized that tool was just what I needed to get me through my own struggles.

To survive, Scott relied on his survival training. In that training, he'd been taught to focus on doing everything he could to survive/ thrive for one hour at a time. In other words, if it's 10:22 a.m. where you are, all you have to do is your very best until eleven o'clock. You don't have to worry about picking up the dry cleaning tomorrow, getting all the supplies for the meeting next Tuesday, or what might happen thirty years from now. You only have to focus on doing your very best in this hour.

It's a simple idea, but it has changed my life and I often recommend this technique to friends, family, and clients. Anytime I feel like I can't take another step or that I'm running short on hope, I refocus on "just doing my best for this next hour." For me, focusing on "right now" allows me to live each moment of my life fully awake and aware. Over the years I've come up with a way to help describe this powerful idea using the acronym FAITH.

FAITH = Fully Alive in This Hour

- Fully: Be present with your whole heart and soul. Don't think about what happened yesterday or what might happen in the future.
- Alive: To be awake, to use your senses to their fullest potential. Don't waste this moment. Touch it, taste it, smell it, hear it, see it, live it completely.
- In: To be present, here and nowhere else.
- This: Now.
- Hour: A limited time. You don't have to be fully focused and aware at any other time but this hour. That's all.

PART FOUR

TAME YOUR ANXIETY

Taming the mind is the path to happiness.

—The Dalai Lama, head of state and spiritual leader of the Tibetan
government and author of *The Art of Happiness*

CHAPTER 26

Just Breathe

Slow breathing is like an anchor in the midst of an emotional
storm: the anchor won't make the storm go away,
but it will hold you steady until it passes.

—Russ Harris, physician, therapist,
and author of *The Happiness Trap*

I N THE wellness center where I worked, there's a small sign in the corner of the restroom that says "BREATHE." Just one simple word. But when I came back to work after finishing chemo for leukemia, I was often so tired I wondered how I was going to get through the day. Day after day that sign reminded me exactly how I was going to find the grace and energy to be present for myself, and my clients, all day long.

"Breathe." Just breathe.

That was enough to see me through the day.

I've learned from tough life experiences that deep, focused breathing can soothe anxious feelings, give you strength, and bring peace to the darkest corners of your life. The daily practice of meditative breathing offers a reservoir of stillness you can access in the midst of any crisis or trauma.

This practice can be particularly helpful for women who suffer from panic disorders. Women are more likely than men to have respiration-related symptoms, and deep breathing can be a powerful way to ease those symptoms.

How You Breathe Makes All the Difference in How You Feel

We're not talking here about the shallow, rushed breathing we tend to do as we race from place to place, desperately trying to get everything done. We're certainly not talking about the nervous, hurried breathing we often do before tackling some anxiety-provoking challenge.

We're talking about relaxed, rhythmic breathing that calms the body and the mind. This type of breathing sends a message straight from your respiratory system to the part of your brain that stimulates your parasympathetic system, (This is the calm, cool, and collected part of your nervous system. The other part of your nervous system, the sympathetic nervous system, gets your body ready for both physical and mental activity.)

The following techniques are arranged in order of when to use which technique, starting with breathing exercises to use when you're in the middle of a panic attack and moving on to methods that are more useful for dealing with long-term anxiety.

Use in Case of Panic

For that "My hair is on fire," "I'm having a panic attack," or "I'm scared out of my mind" feeling, I recommend the following two breathing techniques.

CO$_2$ Rebreathing

This first method is called CO$_2$ rebreathing The jury is still out on the research on rebreathing, but this method works for me.

To "rebreathe," cup one or both hands loosely around your mouth and slowly breathe in and out through your nose until you feel calmer. That's it.

This breath works to rebalance your oxygen and carbon dioxide levels. And while it may not always stop a panic attack, I find it can reduce the severity of your symptoms.

Shoulder or Shrug Breathing

The other technique I find useful for panic and other highly emotional situations is a breathing technique I call either shoulder breathing or shrug breathing.

I love this technique because it's easy to explain, easy to do, and really effective.

A shoulder breath is exactly what it sounds like. As you inhale, lift your shoulders as high as they'll go. Feel free to exaggerate the gesture. Then exhale with a whoosh and let your shoulders fall into a relaxed position.

As you breathe in, you may notice that your body tenses. As you breathe out, feel the relaxation spread throughout your body.

I like to imagine as I exhale that the bones in my body suddenly melt and I feel boneless. That's the feeling we're going for here.

Give it a try and see what happens for you.

For Ongoing Relaxation and Creating a Center of Calm

The next few breathing methods are great to use in the moment, as well as throughout your day, to create a sense of peace and ease. You can do them in the morning before you get up, at night after you climb into bed, in the car, on the way to work, or before that big meeting. Best of all, the more you do them, the calmer you'll feel.

Soft Belly

I first read about the soft-belly technique in James S. Gordon's book *Unstuck: Your Guide to the Seven-Stage Journey out of Depression*. I have since shared it with friends, family, and clients with great success.

Dr. Gordon suggests you begin the soft-belly breath by finding a quiet place where you can be alone for a few minutes, surrounded with things you love or that bring you comfort or peace. (I think that's a wonderful idea for any kind of solitary breathing or meditative practice.)

The next step is to sit, get comfortable, and begin breathing. Gordon recommends breathing in through your nose and out through your mouth, and I'm sure that works for most people. (So go ahead and try it his way.) But for this kind of breathing, I find it less distracting to breathe in and out through my nose. Experiment and see what works for you.

As you breathe out, let your belly go soft. Feel your entire body relax.

Gordon recommends you concentrate on the word "soft" with each inhalation and the word "belly" with each exhalation. I think that's a great way to get started with this kind of breathing. I encourage you to take this a step further and find focus words that help you create a deepening feeling of calm in conjunction with your breathing practice.

I often focus on the word "let" as I inhale and on the word "go" as I exhale. You can use those words or come up with words that have power and resonance for you. For instance, you could focus on the word "love" or "peace" as you inhale and the word "surrender" or "soften" as you exhale. Be creative as you explore the language for words that can help you feel calmer, more centered, and loving.

Coherent Breath

Now let's add another type of breathing to your anxiety-calming tool kit.

This breathing technique builds on the soft-belly technique and comes from the book *The Healing Power of the Breath* by Richard P. Brown, MD, and Patricia L. Gerbarg, MD.

The idea of this technique is to slow your breathing to three to six breaths a minute, which will probably feel slower than usual at first. But if you stick with it, it will soon feel natural and easy.

I do this breath by counting slowly to five as I inhale and counting to five as I exhale. As you give this breath a try, I encourage you to experiment with the counts. You may find breathing in and out to the count of four or six works best for you.

Once you find a rhythm that's comfortable for you, you can deepen your relaxation by finding five focus words you can repeat as you inhale. Then find a five-word focus phrase to repeat as you exhale. For instance, try "I now breathe in peace" as you inhale and "I let go of stress" as you exhale.

As always, this is *your* practice, so feel free to use my words, find words that resonate with you, or stick with the counting. As long as what you're doing feels good, you can't do it wrong.

If you're having trouble slowing your breathing down or you find you could use some guidance to keep you on track, Brown and Gerbarg's book comes with a CD that leads you through this breath and other breathing practices.

Resistance Breath

Brown and Gerbarg's resistance breath can bring a sense of calm to your day and can be used to ease panic. In fact, I find the resistance breath the most calming of all these techniques (in spite of its name). I find it easy to do. I can do it anywhere and at any time. Try it and see how it works for you.

To begin, breathe in through your nose to a count of five (with a soft belly). Then purse your lips. (I do this with as little effort as possible and move my lips to make as small an opening as possible, but do what works for you.) Now exhale to the count of five. (Or use your five-word or five-syllable phrase from above.)

I've discovered that how you exhale changes the effect of this technique. If you breathe out with a whooshing sound, this breath brings instant relaxation and makes it useful for dealing with panic. When you exhale with a more controlled breath, I find this breath works well as a long-term technique for building a center of calm into your life. Try them both and see which works for you.

Again, this is a breath you can use when you need to calm yourself. You can use it on its own or you can use it in conjunction with the coherent breath. You can do one kind of breath ten times and then switch to the other for ten repetitions.

Like the techniques above, you can do this as many times as you need to feel relaxed.

Breath Moving

Brown and Gerbarg's breath moving works exactly the way it sounds, and I find it fun and energizing after a long day.

Here's how it works.

Relax and breathe in as you count to five. Then breathe out as you count to five. Once you've established a comfortable rhythm, begin to imagine with each inhale that you're sending your breath to the top of your head. Can you feel it there? What does it feel like?

As you exhale, imagine that breath is now flowing to your tailbone. Can you feel it moving through you? Does it flow freely? Can you feel your body relaxing as the breath swirls around your organs, soothing them and easing any tension? If you like, you can include a focus phrase or focus word to help you relax more deeply.

Repeat this cycle for as long as feels comfortable. Then, if you're ready to try something new, inhale and send your breath all the way down to your feet. Does that feel different? Does it feel better? Is it harder to do? Does it feel more relaxing?

I find the breath-moving technique most useful after a long, physically challenging day. There's something really soothing about imagining the breath moving through the body that can relax you physically as well as emotionally.

Make Them a Part of Your Day

I've given you some of my favorite breathing techniques. I hope you've tried some of them, and if you missed any, you're welcome to come back another day and give them a shot.

The CO_2 rebreathing, shoulder/shrug breathing, and soft-belly breathing are great for panic and emergencies. Soft belly, the whole or comprehensive breath, and the resistance breath are fine for using on the spot, but when used as a daily practice, they can create a foundation of calm in your daily life.

CHAPTER 27

Meditate

The quieter you become, the more you can hear.

—Baba Ram Dass, spiritual teacher, psychologist,
and author of *Be Here Now* and *Walking Each Other Home*

MEDITATION quiets the mind. The practice of slowing the body and turning your focus inward allows you to connect with the deep, mysterious part of you that knows you have no reason to hurry, worry, or doubt. In the same way physical exercise brings strength and an ease of motion to the body, meditation brings strength and an enduring sense of calm to your mind.

Research has shown that meditation lowers blood pressure, decreases heart rate, slows breathing, and reduces anxiety, especially in women. A recent study done at Brown University found that meditation was more effective in helping women feel better emotionally than men. So it's no wonder we're more likely to use meditation to calm ourselves. And here's the best news of all: Another study found menopausal women who used meditation reduced their hot flashes by 39 percent. Many women also report that meditation can be particularly helpful during pregnancy and birth.

So if you're interested in starting a meditation practice of your own, here are a few types of meditation for you to explore. Please feel free to try one or all of them.

> Meditation should always feel good. If anything about the process is uncomfortable, stop. And if you have symptoms of a serious mental condition, depression, or trauma, I recommend you try meditation only under the guidance of an experienced professional.

Traditional Meditation Practice

Here is one way to practice meditation.

Begin by choosing the focus point of your practice. That focus point can be:

- The repetition of a single word or phrase or sound
- How and what you're thinking
- How you're feeling emotionally
- How your body feels
- Your breath as it comes in through your nose, then goes back out through your nose

If you choose to focus on a word or a phrase, I recommend you choose something that resonates with you. As you inhale, you might use the phrase "I am at peace" or "I breathe in peace." As you exhale, try the phrase "I now go deeper" or "My peace now deepens."

You might also want to consider bringing your attention to this quote by the Vietnamese monk and author Thich Nhat Hanh: "Breathing in, I calm body and mind. Breathing out, I smile. Dwelling in the present moment, I know this is the only moment." See what works for you.

Step One: Once you've chosen your focus point, sit or lie in a comfortable position in a place where you aren't likely to be disturbed. Close your eyes. Then allow your body to relax, starting at the crown of your head and working down to the soles of your feet.

Step Two: As you begin to breathe more deeply, gently bring your attention to your focus point with each inhale and each exhale. If any stray thoughts intrude, notice them, then allow them to drift away like a leaf swirling away on the current of a peaceful river . . . Continue as long as you feel comfortable. In the beginning that might be only a few minutes. But if you're consistent with your practice, you'll find you can work up to fifteen or twenty minutes in just a short time.

For meditation to be effective, it's important to show up for practice at least once a day. Most women find it works best to meditate in the morning before breakfast, but meditation will work whenever you can fit it into your day. The trick is to be consistent in your practice.

If you want some help in getting started, you may want to look for a good meditation class in your area. Many women find connecting with others makes meditation easier and more fun.

Visualization or Guided Imagery

The other type of meditation I often use with clients is visualization or guided imagery. Visualization is a sensory-filled daydream we can use to give us a break from the stress of daily living, to work through problems, or to ease anxiety about the future.

If you've ever gotten lost in a daydream or found yourself wondering what it would be like to walk the red carpet, win an Edgar, or spend time in outer space, then you're already using visualization to help shape your future.

Visualization can also be a way of taking a mental vacation from your anxiety. And like any vacation, just getting away from the daily wear and tear of life can make you feel better all over.

Visualization Practice

Let's begin by looking at how Brenna used visualization.

Eighteen months after her bitter divorce, Brenna felt angry and lonely and was terrified of making the same mistake again. Her friends were urging her to get out of the house more, try online dating, and "just get back on the horse again." But Brenna was paralyzed with fear and happy to spend her evenings and weekends at home in front of the TV.

When she heard about visualization, she decided to give it a try. These are the steps Brenna took to create her visualization practice.

Step One: Set an intention or goal for your practice. Brenna set the intention to imagine the most amazing dating experiences she could dream up.

Step Two: Find a place and time when you won't be disturbed. Sit and get comfortable. Brenna chose to sit in an easy chair in her bedroom just before bed and made meditation part of her evening routine.

Step Three: Relax your body fully, beginning with your head and working your way down to your feet. As Brenna let her breath deepen, she focused on the words "in" on her inhale and "out" on her exhale until her entire body relaxed.

Step Four: As you begin to breathe deeply, imagine yourself in a beautiful place, one where you feel peaceful and at ease. Brenna imaged herself in a peaceful meadow.

Step Five: Begin to notice things around you. Is there a breeze? Is there music playing? Or can you hear the waves breaking on the rocky shoreline? What do you smell? Cotton candy? Fresh-mowed grass? What do you see around you? Are there birds overhead? Are the flowers blooming or just budding? Take your time and allow every one of your senses to open wide and take in the life around you. Remember this is now *your* world. *You control everything here.* You can make it and unmake it any way you want. If there's something you don't like, change it until you *do* like it.

Brenna imagined herself walking through a meadow of wildflowers, surrounded by dark, snow-capped mountains. The breeze was cool and fresh on her cheeks and she could hear the water of a nearby stream splash over the rocks.

Step Six: Now the fun begins. If you're rushed for time, you can end your practice here. But if you want to use this visualization to calm anxiety about an event or help you envision the life you really want, you're going to stay and play.

Brenna began by imaging herself sitting in a café in Paris with a man who leaned forward to listen when she talked. She imagined sipping wine and later walking together to a flower market, where he bought a beautiful bouquet of her favorite roses. She imagined how the wine would taste, how the flowers would smell, and how wonderful it would feel.

At this point you get to imagine anything you want. You have a magic wand you can use to create any scenario you can dream up. The trick here is to include as many physical details as possible. You're not just imagining this scenario, you're *living in it*, as if you were playing an interactive video game.

You can practice going to the ob-gyn's office without a moment's anxiety. You can imagine that you're striding through the airport without hesitation, looking forward to a stress-free flight to someplace wonderful. Then you strap on your seat belt and enjoy the take-off, knowing you're in charge and will be able to handle whatever happens.

> If any scenario is too frightening to even consider visualizing, please don't. This process should be never be stressful.

You can visualize your body healing itself. You can picture yourself giving a successful speech as the CEO of a company or leading a group of young people in a project to turn vacant lots into playgrounds. This is your moment. Dream big. Have fun. Include the things, ideas, and people that make your heart sing.

Over time Brenna enjoyed imagining herself in all sorts of incredible places—snorkeling in Hawaii, on safari in Africa, watching whales in Alaska. She imagined spending time with all sorts of men. She imagined sparkling conversations, romantic gestures, laughter (lots of laughter), and all sorts of fun. She had a ball dreaming up relationships and situations that had seemed impossible when she was married.

Step Seven: If you like, you can set a timer to bring yourself back to reality. Or you can continue your visualization until you feel the process is complete. When you're ready to reconnect with your body and the world around you, begin by wiggling your fingers and toes. Draw in a deep breath and lift your shoulders. As you breathe out, sigh. Repeat the breath and the sigh as you slowly stretch your body awake.

When you're fully alert, you might want to write down what you just experienced, what you liked about the process, and what you'd like to do differently next time. In that way, every time you use this practice, it will be more effective and fun for you.

After a few weeks of meditation practice, Brenna began to get clarity on what had been missing in her marriage and what she wanted in a partner going forward. She didn't want someone like her ex, who wouldn't let his meat touch his potatoes, spent his evenings on his computer, and thought travel was a waste of money. She wanted someone who listened to her, laughed at her jokes, and loved adventure and travel. And when she realized she could choose differently this time, she began to feel comfortable with the possibility of a new relationship.

The nice thing about visualization is that you can change the images at will, and you can keep changing those images as needed.

You never have to imagine the same thing twice. But if you find something you love to imagine, you can visualize it as often as you'd like. No limits, no boundaries.

When Brenna met Eddie in a Cajun cooking class, she felt an instant connection with his adventurous spirit. She began visualizing what it would be like to spend time with Eddie, and when he asked her to dinner, she was finally able to say yes.

If you're new to the idea of visualization or not sure you can remember all the steps, I recommend finding a guide to take you through the experience for the first few times. You can buy a guided-imagery CD or find one on YouTube. Even better, you could write and record your own guided-imagery scenario. This can be a really powerful technique because you get to choose every detail of your visualization. You get to choose the imagery, the story, and, best of all, the outcome.

Using guided imagery is like going into your own interior studio or workshop, where you get to create what you want and let go of what you don't want. It empowers you to see possibilities and allows you to imagine those possibilities into real life.

So, go, dream.

Other Meditation Techniques

Finally, meditation doesn't have to be something you do in a class or alone in a quiet space. You can bring the practice of meditation into your everyday life by turning your attention outward and by looking at things you do daily in a new way.

Stephanie Vozza recommends some great ways to add mindful practices into your life in her article "Meditation Techniques for People Who Hate Meditation."

Walking Meditation

You may find that taking a walk is a great way to relax physically. If you want to turn your walk into a mindful meditation, all you have to do is choose a mantra/word/phrase to repeat with every step you take. If you like, you can think "left" every time you step with your left leg, and then think "right" as you move your right leg. You can repeat a word like "calm" or "peace" or a phrase or a prayer. If none of that resonates with you, you can just focus on the word "walking" and repeat that with each step.

Physical Motion Meditation

Like walking, any kind of repetitive physical activity can be a type of meditation. You can meditate while you swim, bike, vacuum, or shovel snow. Simply allow your mind to focus on the sensations in your body as you move and feel the sense of calm that comes with mindful meditation.

Mindful Red-Light Meditation

Here's a wonderful way to add moments of calm to what otherwise might be a tension-filled day. When you're stopped at a red light or waiting in line at the grocery store, just bring your attention to your breathing. That's all. Just breathe. I bet you'll find that simple act always brings your focus to the present moment. Then enjoy the sense of peace that comes with that kind of focus.

Eating/Drinking Meditation

I love this one. You can turn any meal or snack or even drinking a cup of tea into a meditation just by taking the time to savor the experience. Chew slowly. Be aware of the way the food smells, tastes, and feels in your mouth. Eat slowly, mindfully. Be present to how the food feels in your body. Be grateful for the way it nourishes you. I like to wrap my hands around a cup of tea and feel the warmth of the liquid. I inhale the steam and the scent of the tea before I take a sip.

Make mealtime an event to be savored, not a chore to be done with.

Task-Related Meditation

Many of the routine things you do every day around the house can be used as a meditation. Folding laundry, washing dishes, slicing vegetables, or even washing your hands can serve as meditation if you slow yourself down and bring your full focus to what you're doing and how you feel while you're doing it.

Meditation is the simplest way I know to build a core of calm into your life. Whatever type of meditation you choose, committing to a daily practice will bring a sense of peace and ease into your life.

CHAPTER 28

Sleep

The best bridge between despair and
hope is a good night's sleep.

—E. Joseph Cossman, entrepreneur and author of *Making It!*

VICKY, forty-eight, had trouble falling asleep and even more trouble staying asleep. Night after night she lay awake for hours, staring at the ceiling, worrying about the pile of unfinished work on her desk, the fight she'd had with her son, and that she probably wasn't going to be able to fit into her jeans if she kept on eating the way she'd been eating. In the morning she'd head off to work, dragging and exhausted. Sound familiar?

According to an article on HuffPost, women are the most sleep-deprived people in this country. (As if we didn't already know that.) Single working women and working women with small children are the most exhausted, but most of us don't get enough shut-eye.

Sixteen percent of us report missing one or more days a week from work in the past month because of sleep issues, and 67 percent of us report having a sleep problem a few nights a week.

Like Vicky, we're trying to get everything done before we nod off for the night. We stay up late answering work emails or treat ourselves to a couple of hours of late-night TV after a hard day. Or maybe we manage to go to bed at a decent hour, but our anxious thoughts keep us awake. We replay that scene with our in-laws or that woman in the drugstore over and over in our minds until the first light of dawn.

And maybe like with Vicky, hormones are playing a role in your sleepless nights. Thirty-three percent of all women report insomnia as a symptom of their PMS. Pregnant women almost always experience sleep disturbances of one kind or another, and 61 percent of us suffer sleep issues during both perimenopause and menopause. Just thinking about it is enough to keep us up at night.

So do you get enough sleep? Are you refreshed when you wake up and ready to take on the new day? Or are you cranky, tired, and on edge as you drag yourself to the breakfast table? Do you need that cup of coffee to make you feel human in the morning? Do you nod off after lunch? Do you struggle to stay awake during the four o'clock meeting?

Scientists are still on the fence about exactly how much sleep we need, but usually your body will tell you exactly what it needs and when it needs it. If you start yawning and are having trouble keeping your eyes open at 10:00 p.m., that's a message from your body that it needs sleep. If you ignore those signals and stay up surfing the web until midnight, your body, brain, and emotions are going to pay a price for not listening. And over time that price can become pretty steep.

The first step in getting enough rest is to start listening to your beautiful body. And when it tells you it needs rest, rest. That means setting a bedtime that works for you and sticking to it, finding a way to work a nap into your day, or arranging your schedule in a way that allows you to give your body the rest it needs.

But what if you go to bed at a reasonable hour every night, then have trouble falling asleep or staying asleep? What do you do about *that*? Let's talk.

Getting to Sleep

There are lots of plans and techniques to help us get to sleep and stay asleep. But this is not a "one size fits all" process. This is a "try everything and see what works best for you" process.

Create a Routine

When my children were young and we were trying to get them to sleep through the night, someone told us to establish a firm, consistent, loving bedtime routine. The child knows what to expect and gets in the habit of going to bed without making bedtime a battleground. It was great advice then, and it's still great advice, no matter how old you are.

Vicky found that a regular bedtime routine let her body and her mind know what to expect. She ate her crackers, took her shower, read her book, and then drifted off to sleep. No arguments, no muss, no fuss.

Get Daily Exercise

If you want to get a good night's sleep, one of the best things you can do during the day is to get some exercise. (See "Get Moving," p. 200.) Regular daily exercise relaxes your body and your mind and is a wonderful way to combat insomnia. The only caveat is not to do any vigorous activity right before bedtime. The body needs time to cool down before sleep. (Although doing some gentle yoga or qigong can relax you and may help you sleep more soundly.)

Avoid Caffeine

Caffeine is a stimulant and can keep you awake for hours after bedtime. If caffeine bothers you, make sure you stop all caffeine consumption by 3:00 p.m. (or noon for some—again, see what works for you). Remember there's caffeine in chocolate, tea, and some over-the-counter drugs, so stay away from them as well as that last cup of coffee. (See "Caffeine," p. 265.)

Make Good Food Choices

What you eat at dinner and throughout the evening can have a big impact on your sleep. For some women, eating too much for dinner can keep them awake into the wee hours. For others, eating the wrong kind of food (fried or greasy food in particular) is sure to cause insomnia. On the other hand, like Vicky, *you* may find that eating a small snack of a couple of graham crackers or a banana may actually help you get to sleep.

Drink Moderately

Drinking too much of any kind of liquid before bed can mean you have to get up during the night to pee, and that can interfere with sleep. But some women swear that having a cup of chamomile tea (or other herbal tea) or a cup of warm milk is essential to their sleep routine. Again, this is going to be up to you.

Avoid Alcohol and Nicotine

Some women rely on alcohol to help them fall asleep. But in her article "Sleep Your Anxiety Away, Part I: You've Tried the Rest, Now Get Some Rest," Becki A. Hein, MS, LPC, writes, "Although you may feel temporarily relaxed after using alcohol, it causes you to wake up later at night, interrupting deep sleep and REM sleep."

So alcohol may help you get to sleep, but it can interfere with the most restful and important part of your sleep pattern. Hein goes on to say, "Nicotine is another stimulant which disrupts sleep, so cut down or eliminate smoking to improve your sleep."

Enough said.

Relax

In addition to thinking about what you're eating and drinking, you may want to consider taking a hot shower or a bath to help you relax and wash away the cares of the day. (See "Bathe in It," p. 253.) Try listening to some relaxing music, reading a few chapters from a favorite book, or playing a CD of bedtime meditations. I really like Louise Hay's morning and evening meditation CD, but there are lots of wonderful choices out there, including my own CD, *Creating a Calm Day*.

Create a Calm Environment

Another step to falling asleep is to make sure your bedroom is exactly the way you need it to be to ensure you drift easily into a peaceful night's rest. It's generally recommended that your bedroom be dark, cool, and quiet, with all electronics turned off—or, better yet, in another room entirely. But I know women who happily fall asleep with the TV or the lights on.

Be sure you have a clean, comfortable bed that supports you in a way that feels right to you. If your mattress is too hard or too soft or has a deep valley worn in the middle, maybe it's time to invest in a new one.

Again, if it's working for you to fall asleep listening to the baseball game or Mozart, great. If it's not, try turning things off for a night or two and see what happens.

While we're talking about electronics, why not consider either charging your phone in another room overnight, silencing the notifications, or lowering the brightness of the screen.

You might be surprised at how these small changes help you sleep.

Finally, you might want to write down all your worries of the day, drop them into a worry box, and leave them there for the night. (See "The Worry Box," p. 268.)

I Still Can't Sleep

So you've eaten a light meal, done without caffeine, gotten your morning walk, and established the perfect bedtime routine for you. You climb into bed at your usual reasonable bedtime and you still can't sleep, or like Vicky, you wake up in the middle of the night and can't get back to sleep.

You lie awake counting the hours until you have to get up, worrying about how you're going to get through the next day without any sleep. You struggle to relax and to quiet your racing mind, but it refuses to cooperate.

Now what?

Begin by remembering you've had sleepless nights before and survived to tell about it. Know that tomorrow will take care of itself, and focus fully on the present.

Allow your body to sink into the bed and see how comfortable you can make yourself. Do you need an extra pillow? Could you open or close a window? Challenge yourself to see how many ways you can find to make your body relax.

Now breathe. Once you're comfortable, try Dr. Andrew Weil's simple, effective breathing technique to help you relax into a good night's sleep:

- Exhale through your mouth.
- Close your mouth and inhale through your nose for a count of four.
- Hold your breath for seven counts.
- Exhale through your mouth.
- Repeat the sequence three times.

To deepen your relaxation, you might try the qigong pose Overwhelmed, Lying Down/Middle of the Night (p. 230) or the Corpse Pose (p. 222).

Ways to Think Yourself to Sleep

Now that you're relaxed, focus on your thoughts. Instead of berating yourself for not being able to fall asleep or worrying about the things you didn't get done this week, why not think about this as an opportunity to enjoy some quiet time all to yourself? Here are a couple of suggestions to get you started.

Pray for or think about others. This isn't for everyone, but even if prayer isn't your "thing," you still might find just thinking about the people in your life can be a peaceful exercise. Here is a practice that works for Jackie.

Begin by picturing one by one the people in your life who are struggling or going through a tough time. Once you have their image firmly in mind, ask that they be given whatever it is they need. If you make it through that list, expand that list to friends and family you haven't seen in a while and continue the process.

You can go all the way back to your childhood if you want or include people in the news who could use a good word.

Relive a wonderful memory. Think back to that day when everything went right. You got the job, finished the quilt, won the prize, climbed in the Alps. Remember the details and the joy of it. Savor it and look forward to all the days ahead of you that will be just as wonderful.

Imagine your perfect life. If your life were perfect, where would you be waking up? What would you have for breakfast? Who would be there with you? What would you have around you? What clothes would you wear? What things would you own? What kind of car would you drive? How would you spend your day? How would you feel at the end of this perfect day?

Problem solve. You can use this quiet time to really think through a problem or worry that's been on your mind. (This is not a worry session. This is an opportunity to look at your concern from a different point of view or ask yourself new questions about finding a solution. The minute you start to worry, stop. Either refocus on solutions or more positive thoughts, or go back and try one of the other techniques.)

Get up. If, after twenty minutes to an hour (depending on how you're feeling), none of these techniques have worked, feel free to get up and do something relaxing for a while. (No reading work emails or anything that's going to make you anxious.)

You can read, try a few easy yoga poses, write in your journal, or brew yourself a cup of herbal tea. The mission here is to distract yourself from your worrying and create a sense of calm certainty that you will soon be able to fall into a deep, restful sleep. Once you feel fully relaxed, climb back into bed and begin to get comfortable again.

If getting up once doesn't work, know that you can get up as many times as necessary. You don't have to lie awake all night suffering. There is always something you can do to help yourself feel better.

CHAPTER 29

Just Say No

We must say "no" to what, in our heart, we don't want.
We must say "no" to doing things out of obligation, thereby
cheating those important to us of the purest expression of our
love. We must say "no" to treating ourselves, our health, our
needs as not as important as someone else's. We must say "no."

—Suzette Hinton, singer, musician, actress,
and author of *The Sound of my Life*

WHEN PETRA opened her own catering business, she
was excited about finally being her own boss. She thrived
on the hard work. She took every job that came her way.
She worked ten-hour days and sometimes worked seven days a week.
Her business thrived, and soon she was able to hire two assistants to
help her keep up with the workload. But at the end of her first successful year in business, she found herself anxious, exhausted, cranky,
and thirty pounds heavier.

She told Helen, a local farmer who supplied her with fresh produce, "This is not the way it's supposed to be. I'm miserable, and I have no idea how long I'm going to be able to keep this up. What am I going to do?"

Helen smiled. "You're going to start saying no."

Petra looked at her like she was crazy. "I can't say no. That would ruin my business."

"You can't afford not to," Helen said. "Take it from someone who learned years ago, the only way to make sure both you and your business thrive is to stop living your life to please everyone else. This is your life. Own it. Start saying no to the things that don't feel good or right to you and see how your life changes for the better."

"But if I turn down customers, they'll go to my competition and I won't have any business," Petra said.

Helen nodded. "It may feel like that at first, but I found saying no helped me get rid of customers who weren't working out for me. And in time, I was able to replace them with customers who were much more in line with my way of doing business. At the end of eighteen months, my profits actually went up and I was working fewer hours.

"Limiting my work hours to eight a day and not working weekends helped bring balance back into my life. And once I had more time for myself, I found I had much more energy for my work. Just give it a try, and get ready to feel much better about yourself and your work."

With some support from Helen, Petra started turning down last-minute jobs and jobs that involved too much travel or involved working with customers who were impossible to please. She took two days off every week and never got to work before 11:00 a.m. To her surprise, she started feeling better almost immediately. She felt her sense of excitement and adventure at being her own boss begin to return, and going back to her tap-dance class helped her start to lose weight.

How about you? Are you overwhelmed, overburdened, and exhausted? Do you overcommit because you're afraid to disappoint someone else? Do you say yes when your whole body is screaming no? Me too.

When to Say No: Setting Your Priorities

What finally helped me tackle the challenge of learning to say no was the book *Take Time for Your Life* by Cheryl Richardson.

Cheryl recommends you begin the path to saying no by creating a list of your absolute yeses. In other words, begin by listing your priorities. I know making lists feels like "just one more thing to do," but setting priorities for your life pays off in the end big-time. Even if you have no trouble saying no, being clear about what you value most in your life is essential to creating a great life.

So ask yourself, "What do I really need to do to take care of myself emotionally, spiritually, and mentally? What are my bottom-line needs for a fulfilled and happy life?"

Do you want to spend more time with your family? Do you want to go back to school? Open a boutique? Create a video game? Move to the next level at work? Find a spiritual community? Buy a house?

What do you need to do to create the life you have always dreamed of having?

What do you need to add? What do you need to let go of?

Now that you've given it some thought, write down the things you need to thrive.

Here are my priorities:

1. Physically

2. Emotionally

3. Spiritually

4. In relationships

5. At home

6. At work

7. In my spare time

8. For fun

Now that you've filled in the blanks, you have a solid foundation for building your life around your heart's desires. You also have an effective guide to what you will allow into your life and what you'll want to say no to.

When someone asks you to do something, you can take a minute to check mentally with your yes list. If the request doesn't help you move toward any of your heart's desires, consider saying no.

How to Say No

For most women, this is the hard part. Here are some ways to say no with grace and compassion for everyone involved (especially you).

Think before you speak. My favorite technique for dealing with requests is to ask for time to think them over. By giving yourself some extra time to think, you give yourself the opportunity to check in with your priorities and your schedule and maybe even talk things over with a trusted friend before making your decision.

This works on two levels. First, you're not resentful about taking on a task that becomes a burden and takes time away from your priorities. Second, when you say yes, it means you're tackling this task because you want to, not because you were guilted into it.

Be brief, concise, and honest. For instance, "Thank you so much for asking me to _____, but I'm afraid I'm already overcommitted at work/home and I don't think I could give it my best effort. I'm sorry and hope you'll understand."

Don't offer long apologies or complicated explanations. If the asker asks again, simply repeat yourself until your message is clear and he/she stops asking.

Practice. It can really be helpful to decide in advance what you want to say and then rehearse how you're going to say it. You can practice alone or with a trusted friend until you feel comfortable with the words and any fear that comes up for you as you say them.

Be firm. Be sincere. Apologize if that's appropriate, but this is no place to be wishy-washy. No means no.

CHAPTER 30

Slow Down

We do not want to put pressure on ourselves, or rush ourselves,
because that means we are causing our adrenal glands to release
the hormones adrenaline and cortisol. It is the release of these two
chemicals into the brain that makes us feel "anxious" or "afraid."

—Aaron O'Banion, editor of *Overcoming Social Anxiety*

L ATE ONE afternoon, Sarah was sitting in her minivan waiting
for the light to change. She was worrying about what to have
for dinner and how she was going to meet her payroll for the
month, so she didn't notice that the light had turned green until the
car behind her honked. When she looked up, Sarah realized she had
no idea where she was or where she was going. She panicked until
she noticed her daughter and three of her teammates sitting in the
back of her van all wearing their soccer uniforms. *We're heading for*
the practice field, Sarah thought with relief and worried, yet again, that
she might be losing her mind.

Has anything like that happened to you? Are you so busy and exhausted that you sometimes forget why you walked into the kitchen or why the heck you're standing in the middle of the attic with a roll of plastic wrap? Do you ever worry you're losing your mind? The answer may be that you simply need to slooow down . . .

You know the old expression "Haste makes waste"? Well, haste also makes us upset, cranky, short-tempered, and really, really anxious. Think of how you feel at the end of the day when you didn't get to half of your to-do list. Remember the time you were late to an important appointment, or the time you forgot to pick up your child, or the afternoon your schedule called for you to be in two places at the same time?

Are you getting anxious just reading about the overscheduled, fast-paced life so many of us are living today? Even if you're lucky enough not to be living at such a breakneck speed, are you *really* taking the time to enjoy your work, your family, your friends, your downtime?

Slowing down allows you to enjoy what you're doing. Better yet, it allows you to really savor this short, amazing life, instead of sprinting toward some ever-moving finish line. When you eat slowly, you can actually taste your food. When you take the time to breathe deeply, you can actually smell the newly turned earth in a spring garden and the cinnamon in the cider in the fall. When you slow down and listen to your sister, you might hear the concern in her voice or be able to share a memory.

Slowing down allows you to feel more in control of your thoughts and actions. Slowing down physically cuts down on accidents. Driving more slowly does, too. Whether you're walking or driving, moving to the "slower lane" may keep you safer and will definitely keep you calmer and feeling more in control.

When you slow your thinking, you're better able to think things through. That leads to making better, more-reasoned decisions. Slowing down also helps you focus more quickly and more effectively on the task at hand, which makes you more productive.

How to Slow Down

In her article "How to Reduce Stress by Doing Less and Doing It Slowly," Toni Bernhard recommends four great techniques. Try them all and see what works for you.

1. Figure out how long things really take.

Let's get honest. Do you cheat yourself of a sense of calm by promising to finish things in an unrealistic amount of time? It's time to start telling the truth. Stop pretending you can get to work in forty minutes when you know it takes an hour. No more promising to have the house clean or the report done in an hour when you know it takes twice as long. When you lie to yourself and others about how long things actually take, you guarantee a stress-filled, anxious life.

Write down how long you *know* it takes (not how long you wish it took):

To get to work

To clean the garage

To write the report

To answer the texts and emails

To get through other daily tasks

2. Now that you know exactly how long it's going to take you, give yourself some extra time to get it done.

What if you allowed yourself ten minutes extra to finish each task? What if you were honest with your boss, partner, or children about how much time things are really going to take and what you can and can't do?

What if you committed to "underpromise and overdeliver" as you went through your day? What if you automatically doubled the time you know it's going to take to travel to your destination? If you allowed yourself that extra time, how would you feel about dealing with traffic jams, late trains, and unexpected bad weather?

Would your stress level look different if you included a cushion of time around all your projects? Would you feel less stressed?

3. Consciously perform tasks in slow motion.

This is about focus, breathing, and allowing yourself to relax into an easy, unhurried flow.

If you have trouble slowing yourself down, try my simple four-part technique to transition from overdrive to a state of calm. I like to think of it as a way to push the pause button before shifting from fast-forward into a peaceful slow motion.

- Touch: Tap your lips or chin up to seven times to help you to first focus and then relax.
- Blow: Inhale slowly, then exhale in one great big whoosh. As you blow out, feel your shoulders soften and relax.
- Let go: Repeat the touch and blow until you begin to feel your entire body and mind relax.
- Feel the flow: As you relax, tune in to the rhythm of your body. Chances are it's settling back into its usual slow, steady pace. Without your mind yelling at it to go faster, do more, and stop complaining, your body can relax into its natural peaceful state of being.

4. Do one thing at a time.

For me, this is easier said than done. I listen to music as I write. I watch the news while answering emails, and I'm guilty of cooking while I'm on the phone. How about you? When and where do you multitask? What does it feel like when you're doing several things at a time?

I know when I'm multitasking I'm much more likely to make a mistake. I tend to put the eggs in the wrong dish and press send before I mean to. How about you?

I don't know if it's possible to do one thing at a time in this gadget-oriented world, but what if you committed to doing at least three things a day with your full focus?

What if you decided you would eat dinner without having any distractions—just dinner and maybe some conversation—no TV, emails, texts, or tweets??

What if you turned off all your electronics while you walked with your friends or your children?

What if you sat down and wrote that report without interruption or distractions? What do you think might happen? Do you think you might be more effective?

It all comes down to the quality of your life. If you continue to speed through your days, you'll miss the beauty all around you. If you continue to overbook, rush frantically to get it all done, and put your own needs on hold while you check off the stuff on your to-do list, you're going to miss the joy and beauty around you. We only get one chance at life. Why not make the most of it?

CHAPTER 31

Anchoring

All you need is one safe anchor to keep you grounded
when the rest of your life spins out of control.

—Katie Kacvinsky, teacher and author of
Awaken and *Middle Ground*

HAVE YOU ever watched a young child snuggle with her beloved blanket or favorite stuffed animal to comfort herself? That's anchoring. Have you ever carried a lucky penny or a four-leaf clover? Again, that's anchoring. It's something we all do every day.

Does the smell of baking apple pie bring back memories of your grandmother's kitchen? How would you feel if you saw pictures of your first school? Would you be nervous, excited? What about hearing a song that reminds you of your first love? Might you feel that heady rush of attraction? Would your palms sweat?

All of these things are anchors—a sensation, a touch, a taste, an object, a smell that connects this moment with something in your past and causes you to feel the same emotion you felt in the past.

Anchoring works to change the way you *feel* by changing where you focus your *attention*. In other words, instead of allowing your thoughts to dwell on how scared you are to ask for a raise or to travel on your own, you switch that focus to a carefully chosen memory. And recalling that memory and the emotion that goes along with it can actually *change the way you feel.*

If you think back to a time when you were calm, powerful, and centered, you can actually begin to feel calm or powerful in the present moment. Let's try it.

Take a moment and think of something you're afraid to tackle. Let's say there's a difficult text you've been putting off writing. Imagine yourself looking at your phone, fingers on the keyboard. Can you feel the fear?

All right. Now think back to a time when you felt successful—the afternoon you won the spelling bee or the day you finished the 5K. Remember the details. What were you wearing? How did you feel? Can you feel those feelings now?

As you shifted your attention, did your emotions change? Did you feel better about yourself? Do you feel ready to write that email now? That's anchoring.

You can use anchoring to soothe yourself through a panic attack, to calm yourself before a challenging event like a big exam, or to just plain feel better throughout the day. Once you've created your anchor, you can use it anywhere, anytime you want.

So how does anchoring work?

The Five Steps to Anchoring

Rebecca had a fear of speaking in public. When her boss asked her to fly to Houston to make a presentation to a potential client, Rebecca was terrified. She tried to talk her way out of it, but when she realized her job was on the line, she decided to try anchoring to help her conquer her fear. Here are the steps Rebecca took to successfully face that fear.

Step One: Recall a time, place, or event when you felt calm, strong, and focused. Choose a memory that floods your heart with joy, peace, and love. If you can't think of a memory that has the impact you're looking for, go ahead and make one up. Dream up a scenario that creates the emotion in you that you want to anchor. Be bold. Go big. Have fun.

Rebecca chose to remember a morning walk along the beach on the last day of her vacation.

Step Two: Once you've remembered or created a scenario that resonates with you, take a few minutes to really put yourself in that picture. Look around. Use all your senses.

What do you see? Who's there with you? Are you indoors or outdoors? What colors do you notice? How does the light fall? Be as detailed as possible about what you see.

What do you smell? Can you smell roses blooming? A loved one's perfume? Frying onions? The dusty smell of an attic?

What do you hear? Children laughing? Can you hear the rumble of a subway? Music playing? The clink of a fork against a plate?

What can you taste? The tang of salt air on your lips? The taste of a ripe peach?

What can you touch? Can you feel the rough fabric of an old sofa against your skin or the bark of a tree as you lean your back against it?

Give yourself a few more minutes to experience the *emotion* of this memory and to fully connect with it. Let yourself get lost in the feel of your memory and the depth of your emotions. How does the perfume make you feel? What emotion does that taste or that song bring up in you? If you can, give that emotion a name. Are you peaceful, powerful, joyous? The more you allow yourself to explore this experience with *all* your senses, the richer the memory will become.

Rebecca spent time bringing that morning on the beach to life in her mind. She remembered that the sun was just peeking up over the horizon and the sky was lit with a soft pink and gold light. The waves moved in a soothing rhythm as the tide slowly rose. The wind was off the water and smelled of salt. She'd walked the beach, her feet sinking into the sand. She remembered feeling a deep sense of peace and power and wishing the moment could last forever.

Step Three: Now you need to come up with an anchor that's going to remind you of this moment. Again, this is going to be your choice. You want something that's perfect for *you*. Your anchor can be as simple as a hand gesture or motion. For instance, you can choose to touch the tip of your index finger to the tip of your thumb to make the OK sign, or make a fist, or make any other gesture that suits you and can easily be remembered.

You could use a bracelet or a ring that has some meaning for you. You could wear a rubber band around your wrist as an anchor. It's up to you. Rebecca bought herself a beautiful silver necklace with a single seashell to remind her of her morning on that beach.

Step Four: Once you've chosen your anchor, the next step is to reconnect with your memory. Feel those positive emotions as you touch or create your anchor. Remember the time you walked on the busy city street, heading for dinner with your beloved. Picture the lights, the shape and color of the architecture, the people around you, talking and laughing as they went. Hear the sounds of traffic and the shout of a street vendor selling pretzels. Smell the garlic as you pass a corner restaurant and the exhaust as a bus pulls in beside you. Remember every detail you can. Remember the way you felt that evening as you connect with your anchor.

Repeat this step as often as necessary to make a strong connection between the memory and your anchor. The stronger and more positive emotion you feel, the stronger the link between the memory and the anchor.

Rebecca connected with her anchor every time she practiced her speech. She made a ritual of touching it and imagining herself in her peaceful place of power before she began speaking.

Step Five: The final step is to test out that connection. Make sure it's strong, dependable, and available whenever you need it. Go ahead and give it a try. Can you access the memory quickly and easily? Did you connect with those powerful, soothing feelings? Great.

Rebecca practiced as often as she could. The more she connected with her anchor, the better she felt. And eventually she found she could calm herself by just touching her necklace. Using that anchor to find a sense of calm and power within helped Rebecca make a successful presentation and get over her fear of speaking in public.

CHAPTER 32

Do One New Thing

Never be afraid to do something new. Remember, amateurs
built the Ark; professionals built the Titanic.

—Author unknown

ONE New Year's Eve, I made a resolution to do one scary
thing every day for a year. It didn't have to be big, like leap-
ing out of an airplane, quitting my job, or applying for a real
estate license. It could be as simple as making a medical appointment
or having a tough conversation with a friend, but it had to be scary
enough to make my palms sweat. It sounded like the kind of challenge that would change my life, and I was excited about taking it on.

The only problem was, there were only so many really *small* scary
things I could tackle. By the second week, I was fresh out of the easy
things and was facing only *big* scary things. I felt overwhelmed and
more than my palms was sweating.

I was too scared to move forward, so I quit.

As I look back on that resolution, I can see now how I'd set myself up to fail. By resolving to do something *big* and *important*, I'd scared myself into inaction and a sense of failure that was hard to shake.

How about you? Do you make sweeping promises to change at New Year's, or in September, or just before you have to wear a bathing suit? What happens? Do you make those changes, or like me, do you throw up your hands in resignation and say to yourself, "I knew you couldn't do it. I never follow through on any of my commitments," and then go eat a box of doughnuts?

I swore off resolutions until I overheard someone say they were making a commitment to do one new thing every day for the year. I loved the idea.

First of all, the word "scary" didn't appear in the sentence.

Second of all, I could make the change as big or as small as I wanted.

Third of all, it sounded like *fun*.

Think about the possibilities. You can try a new hair color or go buy yourself a set of new socket wrenches. You can taste a new food, whip up a new recipe, order a different breakfast, eat waffles for dinner, experiment with a new route home from work, wear platform shoes, buy a blouse with puffy sleeves, or no sleeves, eat dessert first, visit a new website, go to a salsa dance class, dance in the moonlight, get up early enough to watch the sun rise, or stay up all night to see the same sight.

You get the idea. You can be as crazy or as uncrazy as you want. You can keep track of your new things or not. You can do it on your own or you can ask others to join the fun.

That year I found a better way to go to work. I learned I like pomegranate juice. I met new friends, visited old friends, and found a great new way to store spices. Not everything I tried was a great success, but that's okay, too. You have to try something before you know whether or not it's right for you.

Here's hoping that trying one new thing might lead you to discover a hidden talent, a hidden strength, or a new and better path to your heart's desires. Here's hoping that knowing you are able to make these small changes helps you feel less anxious, because, truth is, action trumps fear every single time.

CHAPTER 33

Laugh

Laughter is a form of internal jogging. It moves your
internal organs around. It enhances respiration.
It is an igniter of great expectations.

—Norman Cousins, professor, journalist, and author of
Anatomy of an Illness and *Human Options*

First Try Smiling

To change your mood right now, all you have to do is smile. If you don't believe me, give it a try. Go ahead and smile. Not a fake, clown kind of smile, but a real honest-to-goodness grin. Smile with your lips and your eyes and your heart.

Are you smiling? If you are, I bet you feel better. If not, I urge you to give it a try. It doesn't cost anything, and it could change the way you think about how to change your mood.

According to Joseph Stromberg's article "Simply Smiling Can Actually Reduce Stress," published in the *Smithsonian*, studies show what most of us already know: "Smiling can actually reduce stress and help us feel better."

Let's try another experiment. Think of something that worries you or makes you afraid or sad. Take a minute to really let yourself get anxious, fearful, or depressed.

Once you start feeling really miserable, smile with your whole being. How do you feel?

I bet the simple act of smiling lifted your mood.

And here's the good news. No matter what circumstances or challenges lie ahead, you can change the way you feel inside by changing the expression on your face, and that can change the mood of the people around you.

So smile!

Now Laugh

Laughter is a smile on steroids.

Like a smile, laughter lifts your mood, and science now supports what babies and children have always known: laughter makes us feel better all over. Not only does laughter reduce the physical symptoms of anxiety, but it also connects you with the world. The old saying "Laugh and the world laughs with you, cry and you cry alone" turns out to be true. Laughter connects us in a powerful way. If you want to bring people together, make sure they laugh together. If you want to connect with the people around you, laugh with them.

Laughter is contagious. We love to laugh together, which explains those laugh tracks on TV sitcoms. Laughter can ease social situations and smooth over awkward moments. Who knew something so simple could make such a difference?

What makes you laugh? How often do you laugh, and how could you include more laughter in your life? Let's start by looking at what makes you laugh or giggle, guffaw or chortle, snicker or roar.

What books make you laugh? What movies? What YouTube videos? Do babies make you laugh? Puppies? TV shows?

Who makes you laugh? Family, friends, comedians, the woman who does your nails?

Once you have a list of all the things that make you laugh, the next step is easy: *Do more of those things.* See more of the people who make you laugh. Make time to watch funny movies, go to funny plays, and read funny books. Take some time over the next few days to go on a search for all the funny things you can find around you. Make it a treasure hunt for things that make you laugh.

Most importantly, be ready and able to laugh at yourself. One of the best ways to deal with your mistakes and failures, traumas and dramas is to find the humor in them. No matter how difficult the circumstances, when you can find something to laugh at, you gain a different perspective on things. And that new perspective can not only release physical tension and alter your mood, but it can help you come up with a solution you hadn't considered before.

If you feel laughter is lacking in your life and you're looking for a way to get started, I highly recommend laughter yoga.

Laughter Yoga

Laughter yoga is the practice of laughing on purpose. It's based on the idea that purposeful or even forced laughter has the same positive effects on your body, mind, and spirit as spontaneous laughter, and those benefits are available anytime and anywhere you wish.

You can look for a class in your area or watch a laughing yoga YouTube video and enjoy laughing your socks off in the privacy of your own home.

As always, do what feels most comfortable and works best for you.

Here are a couple of laughter yoga techniques from the book *Laughter and Humor Therapy* by Ace McCloud. Go ahead, give them a try. See how quickly a good laugh can change your mood. Remember, you don't have to be in a good mood to make these work. The idea is to "fake it until you make it." The idea is to laugh yourself into feeling good.

Laughter Yoga Techniques

The Stretching Ha's: Stand or sit up tall. Wave your hands over your head and stretch up even taller. Laugh, "Ha ha ha" for a minute or two. That's it. If you like, you can even do it while you're sitting there reading. Just wave your hands in the air and laugh.

The He Ha Ho He Exercise (just the name of this one makes me smile): Again, stand or sit up tall. Put both hands on top of your head. Say out loud, "He he he" to get your laughter juices flowing. Please don't worry if you say "Ha" instead of "He." You can't get this wrong.

Now move your hands down to your chest and shout, "Ha, ha, ha." Next move your hands down to your stomach and yell, "Ho, ho, ho." Finish by stamping your feet and shouting, "He, he, he." If you enjoyed it, do it again.

What could be simpler? What could be more fun? Whether you do laughter yoga alone or with others, it's guaranteed to lighten your mood and lift your stress.

As the great comedian Fred Allen once said, "It's bad luck to suppress laughter. It goes back down and spreads to your hips."

CHAPTER 34

Play

Giving myself permission to PLAY was the cure for my anxiety.
It was a subtle but powerful shift in how I viewed the world.

—Charles Hoehn, speaker, entrepreneur, and author of *Play It Away*

H ere are some pretty serious questions. What do you do for fun? When was the last time you played? What do you really look forward to doing? What fun are you looking forward to today?

If you're like a lot of women, you're probably struggling to remember the last time you did something "just for fun." And you're getting ready to argue that *you don't have time for that kind of nonsense. You're a card-carrying grown-up woman with responsibilities, bills, and a to-do list as long as your arm. You'll get around to fun once you get all the important stuff done, or you'll get to it on your vacation next summer, so stop all this silliness about fun.*

Does any of that sound familiar? How does it feel when you think about a life without fun?

According to Lawrence Robinson's article on HelpGuide.org, "The Benefits of Play for Adults," research shows that play can relieve stress, improve your relationships, and strengthen your connection to others. It can help you feel younger and more energetic, and over time it can even help heal emotional wounds. Best of all, having fun is an excellent way of letting go of the day-to-day worries that haunt us all.

So what looks like a waste of time can actually be an opportunity for you to refocus, realign, relax, and let go of your anxiety for a little while.

There's no goal in play and no point to it, other than to enjoy the heck out of what you're doing. You're not going to be judged on the outcome. You don't have to meet a certain standard of excellence or "do it right." You can't get fun wrong.

Now, let's agree that fun is:

1. Something you really look forward to
2. Something you *seriously* enjoy doing
3. Something you feel great about after you've done it

Fun is not bingeing on cake and ice cream. Fun is not staying up for twenty-four hours playing solitaire. Fun feels good before, during, and *after*. If you feel guilty or have any regrets about what you've done—if you harm yourself or anyone else in any way—*that is not fun*.

Fun is all about pleasure, feeling good, and showing yourself and others a great time. Nothing more. Nothing less.

Which brings me back to my original question. What do you do for fun? Notice I didn't ask what your cousin Merle or your partner does for fun. I asked what *you* enjoy doing. If you're having trouble answering, think back.

What did you love to do when you were a kid? Did you like to color, build models, fly kites, play tag, make puzzles, play dolls, or dance like a happy butterfly? When was the last time you did one of those things? Are you smiling about the possibility of buying a coloring book, at the smell of the crayons or the fun snapping of Legos together? Why not bring that playful fun and that playful spirit back into your life? If you're trying to come up with something that makes your heart jump for joy, here's a list of "Fun Stuff to Do."

Read it over and circle the things that speak to you. Maybe you've always wanted to try jewelry-making or collecting comic books. Maybe you used to do one of these things and would like to get back to it. If so, I am herewith giving you permission to do it again. Maybe there's something you never thought of doing before. Well, why not do it now?

So, let's play.

Fun Stuff to Do

Outdoors

- Take your children to the playground for the afternoon.
- Play tag, hide and seek, or Frisbee. Jump rope, or skip.
- Go to the beach, get in the water, and swim. Splash, dunk, dive under the waves. Be a porpoise. Build a serious sand castle (or one that's not so serious).
- Go for a walk in the rain. Splash in the puddles.
- Play in the snow. Build a snowman. Go sledding or skating. Drink real hot chocolate.
- Plant a garden.
- Create a fairy village.
- Blow bubbles.
- Stargaze.
- Go for a bike ride.
- Fly a kite.

Indoors

- Play a video game (but be careful, they can be addicting).
- Watch a couple of silly animal videos.

- Work on an arts and crafts project just for the fun of it.
- Dance like no one's watching.
- Sing like no one's listening.
- Finger paint (you can use chocolate pudding for extra fun).
- Do a jigsaw puzzle.
- Have an indoor picnic.
- Host a game night. Invite friends and family to play with you.

A Car Ride Away

- Go to the zoo.
- Go play miniature golf.
- Go to an arcade.
- Take your kids to a movie. Get the big bucket of popcorn.
- Go to a toy store and buy yourself that one toy you've always wanted. Play with it.
- Sign up for a pottery class and go get your hands dirty.

Just for You

- Soak in a warm bath.
- Take a nap.
- Get a mani-pedi.
- Get a massage.
- Read something wonderful.
- Take the afternoon off.

At Work

Keep some toys in your desk that you can use yourself or share with others if necessary. Include things like:

- Play-Doh
- A coloring book or two

- Crayons
- Jacks
- A squeeze ball
- A Troll doll
- A rubber nose (for serious emergencies)

Putting Play to Work

Maybe you're thinking, *I'm too busy to add one more thing to my day.* Well, play doesn't have to be something you add to your day. It can be as simple as finding a fun way to do something you're going to do anyway.

Make it a game to see if you can unload your dishwasher before your tea heats in the microwave. See how fast you can clean up after dinner or write a thank-you note. Time yourself and see if you can beat your own record. Keep track, if that feels like fun to you.

Dance in the break room. Hold your business meeting outdoors or at a bowling alley. Try doing a magic trick or two to ease a stressful situation. Wear a funny hat or put on a clown nose. Surprise people. Surprise yourself. When you stop taking yourself and life so seriously, you may well find a new sense of calm and peace in place of your usual worry.

Find friends you play well with. Not everyone is going to want to play the way you do, so look around for someone who's a good fit for your style of having fun. Give your brain a vacation from all that worrying, and let it play as often as possible.

CHAPTER 35

Music

*Just as certain selections of music will nourish the
physical body and the emotional layer, so other
musical works will bring greater health to your mind.*

—Hal A. Lingerman, minister, teacher, counselor, and author of
The Healing Energies of Music and *Living Your Destiny*

YOUR CONNECTION to music began before you were
born. The first sounds you heard were the rhythmic beat of
your mother's heart, the melody of her voice, and the chorus of voices around her. From birth on, you've been surrounded by
music and its incredible power to ease stress and lift your mood.

Listen to Music

Think back to childhood. What kind of music did you listen to?
Classical music? Hip-hop? Blues? Opera? Grunge? Big band music?
Did you instantly fall in love with one kind of music the first time

you heard it? How did that music make you feel? Can you remember a time you used music to change your mood? We can use music to reach our deepest emotions in a way words never could.

As Jane Collingwood writes in her article for Psych Central "The Power of Music to Reduce Stress," listening to slow, quiet music like classical music "can have a beneficial effect on our physiological functions, slowing the pulse and heart rate, lowering blood pressure, and decreasing the levels of stress hormones."

In other words, listening to peaceful music can calm us both physically and emotionally.

Music can also be used to either help you begin a meditation practice or deepen your ongoing practice. Listening to music focuses the thinking part of the brain, leaving the emotional brain free to be mindfully at peace. (See "Meditate," p. 146.)

And now we have some research that tells us that listening to music affects men and women differently. According to Leonard Sax, "Premature baby girls who received music therapy had fewer complications, grew faster, and were discharged earlier than the girls who did not receive the therapy. The research showed there was no effect on the premature boys."

So it makes sense that spending some time each day listening to music may offer women an extra sense of healing calm.

Maybe you're already using music to help you deal with your anxiety. But if not, how could you add some music into your day to create a feeling of calm?

What if you used soothing or inspiring music to ease yourself into your morning? What could be better than starting off your day with music that makes your heart soar or helps you feel cool, and collected?

What if you created a great playlist for your iPod or programmed the perfect playlist to listen to as you drive into work? Do you think you'd arrive at your office in a better mood?

What if you chose to end your day the same way? Instead of watching all the negative stories on the nightly news and going to bed stressed and unhappy, why not listen to music that relaxes you and eases you into a good night's sleep? Ahhh . . .

Make Your Own Music

When she's facing a deadline at work, April heads to the piano in her playroom to bang out "Chopsticks" to ease her tension. Bertha never misses a choir rehearsal. She says she always feels better after singing with her friends. And they're onto something. Studies show that performing music can alter your mood just as effectively as listening to it.

According to Susan Kuchinskas, writing for WebMD, "Casual music-making can short-circuit the stress response, research shows, and keep it from becoming chronic . . . Researchers now know that playing a musical instrument can switch off the stress response, improving physical and emotional health."

And here's some good news: You don't have to be a musical virtuoso to get benefits from playing a musical instrument. You just have to show up and have fun.

So, what about you? Could you hum along with your iPod? Could you sing in the shower? How about performing on karaoke night at your favorite club? What about singing with your children?

What if you picked up that old clarinet or guitar that's been lying in the back of your closet for years and started playing again? What if you joined that a cappella group or garage band like you've been promising to do for years?

Whether you choose to listen to music, to sing, or to pick up an instrument and make your own music, any connection to music will help ease your anxiety and bring a new sense of peace into your day.

CHAPTER 36

Love Your Body

*People often say that beauty is in the eye of the beholder,
and I say the most liberating thing about beauty
is realizing you are the beholder.*

—Salma Hayek, producer, activist, and actress

MARIA WAS fifty pounds heavier than she wanted to be. She hated looking at herself in the mirror. Shopping for clothes was a misery, and she hadn't been on a date in years—because, well, "who'd want to be with a fat girl like me?"

She tried everything she could think of to lose weight—every diet plan that came along no matter how crazy, every new class at her gym no matter how much she hated it.

Every Monday morning she'd get up with renewed determination to lose the weight. She'd weigh herself, groan out loud when she saw the number, and promise herself "this time things will be different." She'd measure her cereal, cut a grapefruit in half, stir flaxseeds into her yogurt, and head for the gym before work.

She'd be "perfect" until Tuesday or Wednesday, when the stresses of her job and her life would catch up with her, and she'd tell herself she needed to pick up a pizza and a soda on the way home, because she deserved a "treat" after working so hard.

Does any part of Maria's story sound familiar to you? Do you struggle with your weight? Or maybe you don't like your nose, your hips, or those flabby wings under your arms, or you're angry at your body for getting older.

Well, if you don't like your body, you're not alone.

A study done by *Glamour* on how women feel about their bodies found that "on average, we have thirteen negative body thoughts daily—nearly one for every waking hour. And a disturbing number of women confess to having thirty-five, fifty, or even one hundred hateful thoughts about their own shapes each day."

Because we don't like our bodies, many of us spend enormous amounts of time and effort trying to look like the perfect images we see all around us on social media. We tell ourselves (and one another) we need to be thinner, taller, younger, firmer, tighter, smoother, fitter, more graceful, agile, or stronger to be "okay."

Over the course of our lifetimes, women will spend, on average, $15,000 on cosmetics, supporting a cosmetics industry that's worth $382 billion globally. And a *TODAY/AOL* body-image survey found that "women spend an average of fifty-five minutes a day working on our appearance . . . That amounts to 335 hours every year—or an entire two-week vacation—lost to their looks."

No question about it, we women are anxious about our appearance in a way most men are not. And I bet you can guess why. It's because we're much more likely to be judged on our appearance than men.

But there's a twist to this you might not expect; at least I didn't. While there's no doubt that men judge women on their appearance, the research reveals that our concern about how we look is also being driven by our *competition with other women*.

Are you as surprised as I was?

And not only are we in competition with one another, but we use that fear of not looking "good enough" to bond with one another. Really!

When we get together, we bemoan our big butts and sagging body parts and wonder about any woman who doesn't join in the self-bashing fest. Just like Maria and her friends.

Every Friday night, they'd meet after work for a drink. Once they'd finished complaining about their bosses, jobs, and lack of a good partner in their lives, the talk would drift to diets, fitness fads, hairstyles, liposuction, gastric banding surgery, where to shop, what to wear, and how to "fix" themselves so they would meet someone new or get that promotion. Then they'd tell one another that things would be great if they "just lost a few pounds."

After years of struggling with diets and bingeing, Maria had just about given up hope that she could ever lose weight, when a friend suggested she join a therapist-led group of women who were also struggling with weight and body-image issues.

Maria was relieved to find the other women in the group were experiencing the same feelings and struggles. From their first meeting, she felt understood and supported. And to her surprise, they almost never talked about food or the numbers on the scale. Instead, the women were encouraged to share their deepest feelings of fear, despair, betrayal, disgust, guilt, anger, and shame. They talked a lot about the self-destructive things they were telling themselves about themselves.

As they explored their negative self-talk, the therapist helped them see that many of the things they were saying to themselves were so cruel they would never dream of saying them to anyone else. In time they realized this self-abuse did nothing to motivate them to take action but, in fact, kept them anxious and focused on failure.

The therapist also helped them see that the way they talked to one another mattered, explaining that public bashing would make the private bashing seem normal and even acceptable, when exactly the opposite was true.

So they agreed as a group that they would speak respectfully to themselves and one another about how they looked and how they felt. No more abuse.

As they continued to explore their feelings, the therapist asked them to make a list of the things about their bodies that they liked. Maria listed her feet, her eyes, her teeth, her strong legs, her long neck, and the shape of her nose. Then, at the therapist's suggestion, Maria and the other women in the group picked one of those positive aspects to focus on every day, throughout the day.

Every time Maria noticed a negative thought about her body, she worked on replacing it with that positive aspect. She stopped scaring herself with threats and insults and started supporting herself with positive affirmations and lots of "attagirls." She worked on not comparing herself to other women and focused on being the best *she* could be. She made and kept necessary medical appointments to keep her magnificent body healthy. She stopped thinking of food as a way to ease anxiety or a way to treat herself and began to think of it as fuel for her beautiful body. She focused on nutritional labels instead of calories. She found a ballet class she really liked and started going on a regular basis. She decided to think of her body as a friend to be respected and treated with tender care. She cheered her successes and acknowledged her failures without judgment.

After a few weeks, Maria started to feel better. With the support of the group, she decided to stop putting off living her life until she lost weight. She bought and wore becoming clothes that fit her well and made her feel much better about herself. She had her hair cut and started wearing lipstick in a color she loved. She joined a bowling league and booked the vacation of her dreams to Paris. Over the next few months, she began to meet new people and even went out on the occasional date.

As Maria changed the way she looked at her life, she found her life changing for the better. As she embraced a healthier lifestyle, she felt a new sense of happiness and self-awareness, and she looked forward to enjoying a slow, sustainable weight loss.

So how about you? Are you ready to make some changes in how you treat yourself?

Ten Ways to Love Your Body

1. If you want to make any kind of change, buddy up. You don't have to join a group or go to a professional to get support, although both those things can help. You can get support from a friend or a family member, or you can partner up with someone online. (Just be sure you have clear goals and guidelines in place before getting started. See "Build a Great Support Team," p. 285.)

2. Use positive self-talk. No more abuse of yourself or others. Start today to change what you say *to* yourself and *about* yourself. Decide to focus not on where you are but on where you're going, and promise that from now on you're going to support yourself by talking to yourself with respect and love. (See "DIY Affirmations," p. 109.)

3. Stop competing with social media images or with women around you. Just be you. Know for sure that you're great just the way you are, without changing a thing.

4. If you're looking for a way to get started, this week go ahead and celebrate every small step you make in the direction of your dreams. Give yourself a pat on the back for even the smallest positive change you make. Do it as often as possible and see what happens. (See "Just Do One Small Thing," p. 122.)

5. Stop putting off living your best life until you weigh a certain number, wear a certain size, or have that brow lift. Celebrate who you are and how you look right here and now. Take time with your appearance. Wear bigger earrings or those boots you've always loved.

6. Treat yourself as often as possible. Have a massage, soak in a sauna, take a long bath, then slather yourself with a soothing body lotion. Take a nap. Sip a cup of your favorite tea. Listen to great music. (See "Music," p. 191.)

7. Record your feelings instead of feeding them. (See "Journal," p. 271.)

8. Get physical. Find an exercise plan you really enjoy and keep at it. Walk, run, dance, or play games with your children. Find fun ways to stay in motion. (See "Get Moving," p. 200.) Check in with your body throughout the day to see how it feels and what it needs, then honor those needs.

9. Focus on eating as a way to fuel your body, not as a reward for working hard or as a recreational pastime. Eat to live—don't live to eat. (See "Eat and Drink This," p. 260.)

10. Forgive yourself for not being perfect. You did your best back then. Now that you're older and smarter, you know more and will do better. (See "The Importance of Not Being Perfekt," p. 89.)

CHAPTER 37

Get Moving

A vigorous five-mile walk will do more good for an unhappy but otherwise healthy adult than all the medicine and psychology in the world.

—Paul Dudley White, cardiologist, advocate of preventive medicine, and author of *Heart Disease*

Why Move?

Our bodies weren't designed to sit at a desk, in a car, or on a subway. We were designed to move. And when we move, we not only get stronger physically, but we get calmer and smarter as well.

Research shows that exercise greatly reduces stress. And here's even better news. An article from the Anxiety and Depression Association of America titled "Exercise for Stress and Anxiety" reports, "According to some studies, regular exercise works as well as medication for some people to reduce symptoms of anxiety and depression, and the effects can be long lasting. One vigorous exercise session can help alleviate symptoms for hours, and a regular schedule may significantly reduce them over time." And here's more good news: *exercise works without any of the side effects of medication.*

So why are 60 percent of women in this country not getting the recommended two and a half hours a week of moderate activity? Because we don't have the time or the energy. Or maybe we've forgotten how much fun moving can be. Or we're thinking of exercise as one more thing on that long list of "stuff to get done." But what if you found some activity you really enjoyed? What if we could find the right exercise plan for you and your lifestyle?

Let's take a few minutes to put together a plan for you that makes moving fun again.

Remember When . . .

Picture yourself in your third-grade classroom. Your teacher is droning on about something boring like pronouns, integers, or the qualities of solids . . . (Please make it something really, really dull.) It's a beautiful afternoon. The sun is shining and a soft breeze is making the leaves dance on the trees outside.

From your seat you have a great view of the playground. There are only ten minutes until the bell rings for recess, and then you'll be free to go outside and play.

If you're having trouble picturing this, make the image your own. Maybe it's seventh grade and you're still listening about those darn integers, pronouns, and solids. In ten minutes you're going to go play tag or hopscotch or ride your bike in the woods.

Maybe you're sitting by a window waiting for the rain to stop so you can go swimming or canoeing. Maybe you're waiting for the snow to start so you can finally get outside to skate, ski, or build a snowman.

Just picture a time in your childhood when you were looking forward to moving.

All right, how are you feeling as you sit and wait for the chance to go play? What are you thinking? Are you dreading it? Are you thinking about skipping it because you have more important things to do? Are you worried that you're not going to be good enough at running, jumping, or skipping or that you'll look foolish if you try?

Or are you looking forward to it? Can you feel that excitement in your body right now as you remember how you used to feel about getting your body in motion? Was there one activity you looked forward to more than others? What was it about this activity that made it so much fun?

What other physical activities did you enjoy when you were a girl?

All right, let's take a look at the last time you "exercised." Maybe it was earlier today, last week, last month, or last year, but think back to the last time you moved your body in a significant way.

What activity/activities did you choose?

Did you feel the same enthusiasm about moving you experienced as a child? (If so, good for you. Feel free to skip ahead to the next section. If not, read on.)

If you're not loving your exercise plan, why not? Is there something about it you could change? Is there something else you'd rather do?

If you don't have an exercise plan or haven't been active in a while, what's been holding you back?

Now let's find a way to move your body that's right for you and your busy life.

Getting Started

Before we move on to choosing the right exercise plan for you, please be sure to check in with your health care provider to make sure you're healthy enough to start any kind of an exercise plan. And, if necessary, let her be a part of choosing the activity that suits you best.

Once you have clearance from your PCP, you can get down to the business of getting your body in motion in a way that eases anxiety and creates a sense of calm in your life.

Lisa goes out for a run when she feels stressed. Molly goes to spin class or yoga. I have friends who hike mountains or swim laps to soothe their body, mind, and spirit. I walk. Walking not only makes me feel better physically, but it grounds me and creates a peaceful center in my life that nothing else can do for me.

I've walked in rain, heat, nor'easters, hurricanes, and snowstorms. I've walked through the miserable side effects of two different kinds of chemo. I walked the day before all five of my surgeries and the week after. I've walked alone, with my family, and with my friends. I've walked in cities, towns, mountains, woods, fields, by rivers, streams, and the oceans on both sides of this country.

I walk every day because I love looking at the sky. I love to watch the way the world changes around me season to season and because walking makes everything in my life better, especially me.

Maybe you walk, too. Maybe you want to try walking. Or maybe walking isn't for you. That's okay. This is about creating a plan that resonates with you. This is about finding ways to get your body in motion that make you feel good.

It doesn't matter what kind of physical activity you choose to do; *what matters is that you do it.* And if you're like most women, sooner or later you're going to stop showing up for an exercise plan you hate. If you don't like to swim—don't. If you don't want to play an organized sport—don't.

If you're not loving your exercise routine or don't have one yet, here's a list of things that will get you up off the couch and moving in healthy new ways.

Take a minute and circle the things on this list you've already tried. Give yourself a pat on the back for those past successes, then circle the items you've always wanted to try. If you don't see an activity listed that you've tried, feel free to add it to the list.

Ways to Be Active

Aerobic machine (elliptical trainer, stair climber, treadmill, etc.)
Aerobics class
Badminton
Baseball
Basketball
Biking
Boot camp
Bowling
Calisthenics
Cardio class
Circuit training
CrossFit
Dance (ballet, hip-hop/funk, Latin, reggae, salsa, tap, etc.)
Fencing

Field hockey
Football
Frisbee/Frisbee golf
Gardening
Golf
Gymnastics
Handball
Hiking
Horseshoes
Housework
Hula-Hoop
Ice-skating
Jazzercise
Jogging
Jumping rope
Kickball
Lacrosse
Marathoning
Martial arts (aikido, judo, etc.)

Pilates
Running
Spinning
Squash
Step aerobics
Stretching
Swimming
Table tennis
Tag
Tennis
Triathloning
Volleyball
Walking
Weight lifting
Yoga
Zumba

Creating *Your* Activity Plan

How many activities have you already tried? Good for you.

Would you want to try them again?

How many activities would you like to try?

Write your top three choices here:

1.

2.

3.

Pick at least one you'd be willing to try and let's get down to business.

Let's agree there's not going to be any more "forcing yourself to exercise because it's good for you." There isn't going to be any more beating yourself up because you didn't do it right, didn't do enough, or didn't do it every day. This is your "no excuse, I'm going to move the way that feels right for me" exercise plan.

Guidelines for Your Exercise Plan

Step One: Once you've committed to an activity, you're going to show up and do it as long as you enjoy it. When you don't enjoy it anymore, you're going to come back here, read this section again, and pick another way to get moving.

Step Two: You're going to start slow and build on your consistent progress. You're not going to berate yourself anymore for not being in better shape. Starting now, you're going to congratulate yourself for having the courage to commit to something new. It's time to be proud of yourself.

Step Three: You're going to forgive yourself if you miss a day. You're going to love your body no matter how you look in spandex. And you are never, *ever* required to wear spandex. If you walk ten minutes today, we're going to cheer for you and look for ten or eleven minutes tomorrow.

Step Four: You're going to stop allowing what you want in the moment to keep you from getting what you really want by asking the following questions:

"How will I feel after I exercise?"

"How will I feel if I don't exercise?"

Step Five: Finally, remember why you want to be more active. Remind yourself that exercise can add years to your life and life to your years. Activity can make you healthier, stronger, thinner, and calmer. It can reduce stress, build confidence, and bring a new sense of empowerment to everything you do.

What would your life look like if you could literally walk away from your anxiety? Why not find out?

CHAPTER 38

Keep Moving, Stay Motivated

A body at rest stays at rest. A body in motion stays in motion.

—Newton's first law of motion

YOU'VE FOUND the right exercise plan for you. You've tried it a few times and it's going well. But research shows women are far more likely than men to say they lack the willpower to make the lifestyle changes recommended by their health care providers. So it's really important to find some extra motivation to keep us moving.

Here are some suggestions to keep you going on cold, rainy days and the days you'd rather have root canal surgery than go to the gym. (You can also use these tips to get motivated in any other part of your life where you want to create change.)

Create a Habit

This one's at the top of the list because it's the most important part of creating any positive change in your life. As Jim Ryun, former politician and Olympic track and field athlete, says, "Motivation is what gets you started. Habit is what keeps you going."

As you may know from past experience, creating a new habit is easier said than done. But today science has stepped in to make this process easier.

In his book *The Power of Habit*, Charles Duhigg explores the latest research about forming a new habit. According to Duhigg, MIT researchers "discovered a simple neurological loop at the core of every habit, a loop that consists of three parts: a cue, a routine, and a reward. To understand your own habits, you need to identify the components of the loops."

In other words, every habit has three parts. When you know what those parts are and how they work together, all you have to do is take out the part that isn't working and replace that part with something that *is* going to work. (I know it sounds a little complicated, but take a look at the diagram on the opposing page. That might help make things clearer.)

Your Routine

So how are we going to put this to work in your life? Let's begin by deciding on the habit you want to create. Let's say you want to go walking every Saturday morning or get to lacrosse practice every Monday and Wednesday night.

Write the routine you want to establish here:

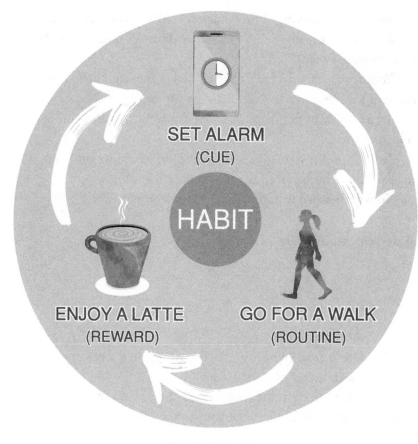

SET ALARM
(CUE)

HABIT

ENJOY A LATTE
(REWARD)

GO FOR A WALK
(ROUTINE)

The Habit Loop

Iris wanted to get up and go to a spin class two mornings a week but was having a hard time getting out of bed. She decided to work on creating a habit to make that class a part of her life.

Your Reward

Now, what reward could you give yourself this week for showing up for that routine every day? What would really make you feel great? A conversation with a friend? Watching your favorite TV show? Reading a chapter in the book you're enjoying? Or do you want to pay yourself for moving? How much would it cost to make sure you show up for your scheduled exercise session? A quarter? A dollar? Five dollars? Twenty?

Your reward doesn't have to cost much, but it should be *something that really inspires you*. It should also be something you know you are willing and able to do for yourself. And you must follow through on your promise.

No fair promising yourself a decaf latte for doing push-ups and then not allowing yourself to enjoy that latte.

So what reward would you like to enjoy this week?

Write your reward here:

Iris decided to treat herself to her favorite reality TV show without guilt for meeting her exercise goals.

Now that we have the routine and the reward in place, all that remains is to create a cue to get you started.

Your Cue

This cue serves as the "on" switch to the "habit loop" and is usually something in your environment that calls you to action.

For instance, you could leave your tennis racket on the passenger seat of your car to remind you to head to the courts. Set the alarm in your phone or have your voice assistant give you a wake-up call. Leave your bathing suit in your briefcase so you remember your commitment to hit the pool after work. Be creative. It doesn't matter what cue you choose. What matters is that it works for you. Again, you may have to try several different cues to find the one that resonates with you.

Write your cue here:

Iris laid out her exercise clothes the night before her class. Then she left her sneakers on the floor by her bed twice a week so she could step into them as she got out of bed. Those cues helped remind her of what she really wanted, not what she wanted in the moment. Over the next few weeks, she started to really enjoy the feeling of working out, and over time she found a number of supportive friends in her class who counted on her to show up.

By the end of six weeks, Iris had a habit in place and she actually began to look forward to her spin class.

Your New Habit

So there you have the three steps you need to take in order to create your new habit. Cue, routine, and reward. Write them in the diagram of the habit loop so you see how *your* loop is going to work.

And remember, if it doesn't work for you the first time out, be patient. Building this wonderful life is going to take time and practice.

Three Ways to Get Motivated

1. Change something. Making a change can be the perfect antidote to exercise boredom. If you like to work out to music, consider downloading some new tunes to inspire you. Upgrade to a better set of clubs or buy new shoes or gloves. Invest in a personal trainer at your gym for a few sessions. If you play a sport, take some lessons to brush up on your skills. The more variety in your routine, the less chance of being so bored that you stop showing up. So be bold. Try something new.

2. Keep track of your successes. You can measure success in all sorts of ways. You can use a mirror, a Fitbit, a pedometer, or an app. But the easiest, most effective way to keep track is to look at how things are going for you in general. Are you feeling better? Do you have more energy? Are you healthier? Are you less anxious, less stressed? If so, then what you're doing is working and you're on the right track. Congratulate yourself and keep on trucking. If not, you know you need to make some adjustments to your plan.

3. Just do it for ten minutes. This is the best trick I know for getting started on anything you really don't want to do. Tell yourself you'll ride your bicycle for just ten minutes or go for a ten-minute walk after dinner. Maybe you'll bike or walk for only ten minutes and that's great. You met your goal, after all. But often you'll feel so much better once you get started that you'll want to keep on doing it. And ten minutes turns into twenty or thirty or more . . . Whether you walk ten minutes or an hour, every step you take brings you closer to that healthy, calm-centered life you deserve.

CHAPTER 39

Yoga

You don't have to be flexible to do yoga. You just have to be willing to shake off the dust and see what happens.

—David Good, wellness expert and yoga teacher

YOU DON'T have to be flexible, young, strong, or in perfect health to get benefits from a yoga practice. You don't have to turn yourself into a pretzel or buy any special equipment or clothes. You just have to show up and do it. And there are lots of reasons for women to give yoga a try.

First of all, yoga has been scientifically proven to significantly reduce anxiety, particularly in women. Just two months of yoga practice can make some amazing changes in your body and bring a sense of ease to your mind and peace to your spirit. Yoga has also been proven to be useful in calming the anxiety and discomfort of PMS. And unlike the medications often prescribed for anxiety, which come with possible side effects and concerns about the need to increase dosages over time, the more often you practice yoga, the stronger and calmer you'll become. So let's get started.

I've taken most of the following postures (asanas) from the book *Yoga as Medicine* by Timothy McCall, MD. This is a great book for any woman who wants to learn how to use yoga for healing.

Alternate Nostril Breathing

This traditional yoga breath is an excellent way to ease stress, anxiety, and even panic. It opens a direct path of communication between the body and the brain, which allows them both to balance and relax. You can even practice this breath in bed at night to relax after a long, hard day. It calms both mind and body and can help you fall asleep. It can also be used to ease a panic attack.

Begin by finding a time and place where you won't be disturbed for the next few minutes. Once you've settled into a comfortable sitting position, shake your hands a few times to get rid of any nervous energy. Place your left hand palm upon your left knee.

Gently press the index and middle finger of your right hand on your forehead, directly between your eyebrows. You're going to use the thumb and ring finger of your right hand to press first your right nostril and then the left.

Using your thumb, gently close your right nostril. Slowly breathe out through your left nostril. Then breathe in through your left nostril. As you lift your thumb, gently press your left nostril closed with your right ring finger. Breathe out through your right nostril and then in through your right nostril. Become aware of how your body relaxes with the outgoing breath. As you inhale, imagine the incoming breath is nourishing your body with new energy and calm.

Continue breathing in and out, connecting with the feeling of fullness on the in breath and the ease of relaxation on the out. If you like, you can add a count of four or five or a focus phrase or word to each inhalation and exhalation to deepen your relaxation.

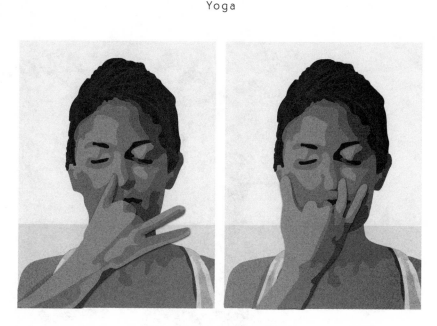

Alternate Nostril Breathing

Continue breathing and relaxing, allowing the inhalation to flow smoothly into the exhalation and the exhalation to flow smoothly back, circling in and out until you are peaceful and calm.

Standing Balance Pose

The Standing Balance Pose is a simple way to calm anxiety. It's easy to do, and you can practice a modified version while waiting in line at the deli or anytime you feel anxious. Begin by standing tall. Then, with one hand, hold on to something solid and stationary for balance and raise the other arm to shoulder height. If you feel strong and have a good sense of balance, you can stretch both your arms to shoulder height. Shift your weight and balance to your right leg, then lift your left foot off the ground just until your weight is on your right leg. Hold for a moment, then return your left foot to the ground. Repeat on the other side.

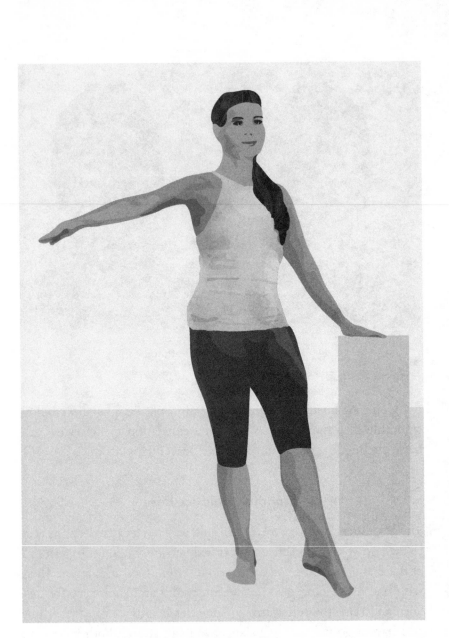

Standing Balance Pose

Tree Pose

The Tree Pose is another powerful pose you can use to create a sense of peace within. It may not sound as simple as the Standing Balance Pose, but if you use a wall for balance, it's just as easy, and it's nice to have a variety of balance poses.

Begin by standing with your right shoulder near a wall. Lightly rest the fingertips of your right hand on the wall for balance. Now, lift your left leg, bending your knee until you can place your left foot on the inside of your right thigh.

If you can't get it up that high, place it just above your knee or on your shin. (Do whatever works best for you. If you feel strong and balanced at this point, try lifting your fingertips from the wall for a moment. If not, enjoy the pose with the wall still supporting you.) Return to your starting position, then repeat on the other side.

Legs Up the Wall Pose

This posture may look odd, and it may *feel* odd when you first try it, but it can be a wonderful way to relax after a stressful day, and you'll reap the benefits of an inverted (upside-down) pose without any extra stress or strain on your body. It can also be safely used in pregnancy.

Begin by folding a bath towel or two (depending on what's most comfortable for you) and have them with you as you sit beside a wall. Lie on your back beside the wall, then swing your legs up against the wall, keeping your hips on the floor but as near the wall as possible. If it would make you more comfortable, slide a rolled towel under your tailbone for extra support, making sure that your weight is on your shoulders and hips. Relax.

You may not be used to being upside down like this, so if you feel uncomfortable, try it for just a few seconds. Doing this posture for only thirty seconds can be useful, and you can build from there.

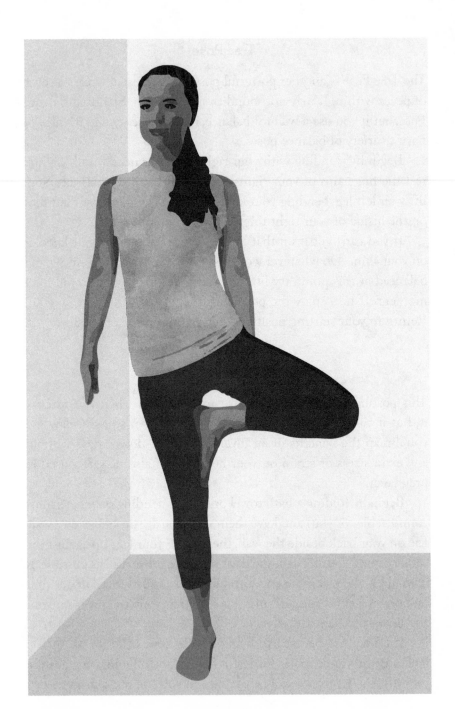

Tree Pose

If this feels too advanced for you, here's a simpler version to try.

Again, begin by folding a bath towel or towels and have them with you as you sit beside a sturdy chair. (You can use any kind of chair, but I find upholstered chairs are the most comfortable.) Lie on your back beside the chair. Swing your legs up over the chair seat, then bend your knees so that your calves and feet are resting on the seat of the chair. Put a pillow under your head for support. Stay here as long as you'd like.

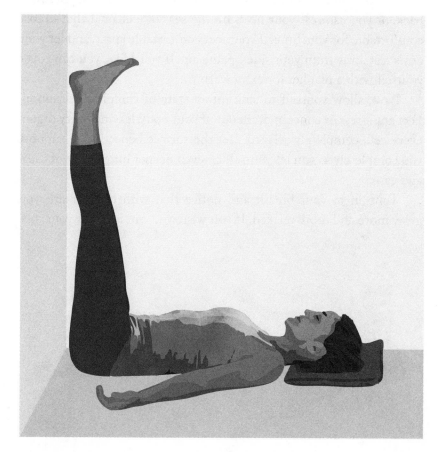

Legs Up the Wall Pose

Corpse Pose

Many yoga classes end with the Corpse Pose, so we'll end with it here as well. But you can do it before, after, or during your practice, or anytime you want to experience deep relaxation. It calms both the body and the mind and can help you fall asleep.

Begin by lying on your back on a mat, rug, or bed or on any comfortable surface. If you wish, you can support your head on a small pillow. You can also add a cushion under your knees to support your back, or you can rest your heels on the seat of a chair if that's most comfortable for you. Spread your feet comfortably apart, and let your arms rest away from your sides, palms up. If you'd like, you can cover yourself with a blanket for extra warmth.

Now, allow yourself to sink into a state of complete relaxation. Feel any stress or concern drain out of your body, leaving every organ, every cell, completely relaxed. Let the surface beneath you support you completely as you let yourself go even deeper into a state of calm and ease.

Tune in to your breath and notice that with each breath you grow more and more relaxed. If you wish, you can imagine your toes

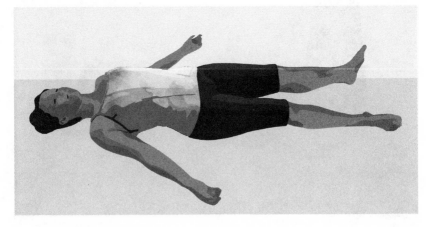

Corpse Pose

relaxing fully, then feel that relaxation slowly work its way up into your ankles, calves, and knees. Feel your hips and spine relax. Imagine your arms and hands growing heavier and feel the peace spread into your shoulders, neck, and head.

Relax fully and remain in this position as long as you'd like. (If you fall asleep, that's okay.) When you are ready, you can wiggle your fingers and toes and slowly come out of the pose.

Let's end with the traditional closing to many yoga classes.

Namaste: "My divine soul recognizes the divine soul in you."

CHAPTER 40

Qigong

Qigong ("chee-GUNG"): a component of traditional Chinese medicine that combines movement, meditation, and regulation of breathing to enhance the flow of qi (an ancient term given to what is believed to be vital energy) in the body . . . The rhythmic movements of Qigong are reported to reduce stress, build stamina, increase vitality, and enhance the immune system. It has also been found to improve cardiovascular, respiratory, circulatory, lymphatic, and digestive functions.

—Taken from medicinenet.com

AT FIRST glance, qigong and yoga look alike. They both use meditation and movement to restore balance and strength to body, mind, and soul. They both can be used to help heal anxiety. But unlike the mostly static poses often associated with yoga, qigong postures are fluid and repetitive.

I find that the repetitive postures make qigong more useful for dealing with anxiety at the moment it occurs, while, in general, yoga is more effective in dealing with long-term anxiety.

Qigong poses can be used to deal with specific concerns like insomnia, fear of public speaking, panic attacks, crisis-worrying, or any hairy, scary challenge that comes your way. And research shows that qigong is particularly useful for managing the symptoms of menopause.

The following exercises are my favorites from the excellent book *Qigong Workbook for Anxiety* by Master Kam Chuen Lam. You can do any of them standing up or sitting down—whatever feels right to you. Try them once or do them as often as you like. You can't get this wrong. (As always, it's important to consult your health care provider before starting any new exercise program. And *if anything hurts, don't do it.*)

For Use When You're Feeling Overwhelmed: Coming Up for Air

According to Master Lam, this posture is useful for any woman who feels overwhelmed with the to-do lists and deadlines of everyday living. And what woman doesn't feel like she's drowning in responsibilities and worry? In truth, this posture is for all of us.

Coming Up for Air calms the body, restores energy, and gives you a feeling of well-being, even in the midst of a crisis.

Begin by standing or sitting in a relaxed position. As you breathe in through your nose, count slowly to six, let your lungs fill with air, and lean back slightly. At the same time, open your arms to the sides, palms open as if you're inviting a wonderful friend or a new experience to come join you. As you move, notice how your body relaxes and the tension around your neck and shoulders eases.

Now, exhale through both your nose and mouth. Let your shoulders relax and bend forward slightly as you release the stress and strain of the day. At the end of that exhalation, let your arms hang

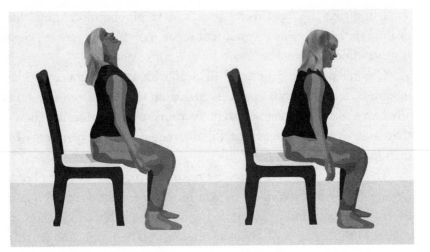

Coming Up for Air

at your sides and your chest muscles relax while you tilt your head forward slightly.

Repeat six times, or until you sense a shift in the way you feel. Continue until calm.

For Inner Calm and Extra Energy: Inner Reservoir

This is a simple way to both calm yourself and replenish your energy in any situation. Lam recommends you do this posture sitting down, but I've found you can do it standing up or even lying down, depending on the circumstance. Do what works best for you.

Begin by relaxing, your arms hanging loosely at your sides. Then slowly move just your right forearm until your right hand covers your lower belly, just under your belly button. Now gently lay your left hand over your right. Be still. Hold the posture a minute or so, feeling your belly move under your hands, letting your body relax fully. Repeat until calm.

That's all there is to this posture, but don't be fooled by its simplicity. This is amazingly powerful, and best of all, almost anyone can do it.

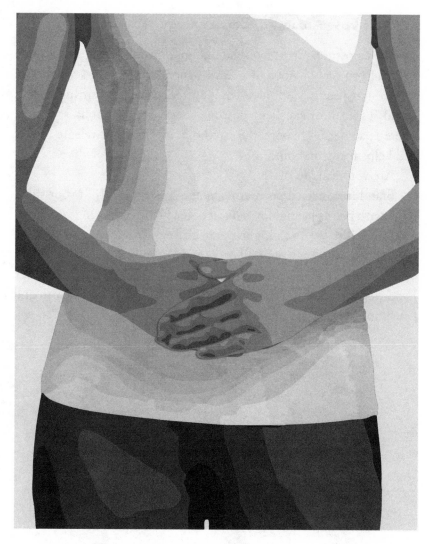

Inner Reservoir

To Ease Anxiety or Boost Energy: Arm Swinging

The next posture, Arm Swinging, is fun and easy and can be done anytime you feel anxious or need an energy boost. It's a wonderful way to start your day or to reenergize after you've been sitting awhile. I find it's also an excellent posture to use before public speaking. There is something about the rhythmic motion that releases stress and helps focus the mind.

Are you ready to play?

Stand in a relaxed pose, arms hanging comfortably at your sides. Now, with palms facing down, fingers gently spread, swing your arms up to shoulder level (no higher, please). Then swing your arms down behind you until they naturally come to a stop.

Continue the swinging motion forward and back, arms parallel, hands relaxed. Feel the solid connection of your feet to the earth and the flow of air through your fingers.

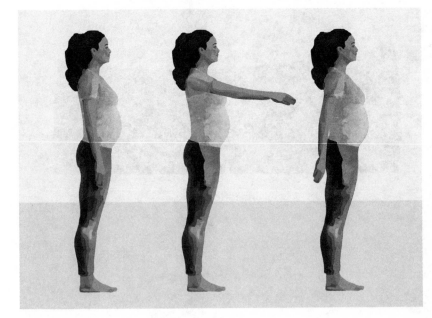

Arm Swinging

You can do this alone, but doing it with your children or other playful adults adds to the fun and can create a healing connection between you. Repeat until calm.

Lam recommends starting with as many repetitions as you can do comfortably and working up to three minutes a day for maximum effect.

To Calm Severe Worry or Panic: Opening the Curtains

This exercise is really useful for quieting worried thoughts or creating a place of calm in the middle of a crisis or panic. I find it can also be used to relax the stress that comes from sitting for a long time. So let's get to it.

"Opening the curtains" is the perfect way to describe this posture. Begin by settling into a comfortable position, either sitting or standing. Now, imagine you're in front of a large window that is hidden behind a pair of heavy drapes or curtains. As you inhale, slowly raise your hands to eye level, palms turned outward as you prepare to spread open the imaginary curtains. Then, as you exhale, slowly push those heavy curtains as far apart as is comfortable for you, remembering to keep your elbows bent, your fingers gently spread. On the

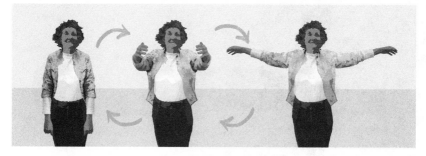

Opening the Curtains

inhale, slowly draw those curtains closed and return to your starting position with your arms by your sides.

If you're standing and would like to add an additional element to this posture, you can lean forward slightly onto the balls of your feet as you draw the curtains open and return to your starting position as you pull them closed. Repeat until calm.

Lam recommends doing this exercise three, six, or nine times. Find what works for you.

For Insomnia, Worry, or an Energy Boost: Overwhelmed, Lying Down/Middle of the Night

I've saved the best for last. This is the best physical technique I've found for dealing with insomnia. You can use this anytime you're having trouble sleeping. You can use it on its own or in conjunction with affirmations, reframing, and/or deep breathing—whatever combination works for you. You can also use it anytime you're feeling overwhelmed, are worn out from worrying, or need an energy boost to get you through the rest of the day. I urge you to try it in as many circumstances as possible and see where it works best for you.

Begin by lying on your back, arms slightly away from your body, palms up.

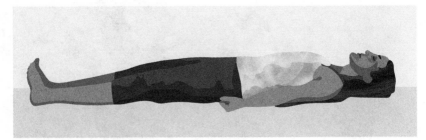

Overwhelmed, Lying Down/Middle of the Night

Now, as you keep your heels on the ground, pull your toes toward your head, feeling the stretch in your calves. Clench your fists and curl them toward your thighs until you feel a tightening in your wrists. At the same time, inhale and lift your head until you can see your toes. Hold your breath a few seconds; then, as you exhale, return to your starting position. Relax. Repeat until calm.

You can repeat this up to six times, but I often find doing it just a couple of times works for me.

CHAPTER 41

Acupressure

*Acupressure is a therapy developed over 5,000 years ago
as an important aspect of Asian, especially Chinese,
medicine. It uses precise finger placement and
pressure over specific points along the body.*

—Andrew Weil, MD, physician, advocate for alternative medicine, and
author of *Spontaneous Healing* and *Spontaneous Happiness*

ACUPRESSURE is, hands down, one of the best ways I know for dealing with acute anxiety, phobias, and panic attacks. Like acupuncture, it works by opening blockages in the energy channels (meridians) throughout the body. Once these blockages are cleared, the body's natural, healing energy is able to flow freely, balancing the body and mind. Like acupuncture, acupressure has almost no negative side effects, and it can be used to heal you both physically and emotionally.

But unlike acupuncture, you can practice acupressure without going to an expert. You don't need to buy any fancy equipment or take a class. You just need to know where the acupoints are and how to massage them.

Acupressure is perfect for emotional emergencies. It's like an emotional first aid kit you can use to deal with sudden-onset anxiety and specific fears (phobias), for instance: the fear of heights, snakes, needles, crowded places, or public speaking. It's useful for panic attacks and even useful in dealing with the fear that you *might* have a panic attack. (How cool is that?)

Of course, acupressure isn't for everyone, and it's important you check in with your health care provider to make sure this kind of practice is right for you.

The following techniques come from the book *Acupressure for Emotional Healing* by Michael Reed Gach, PhD, and Beth Ann Henning, Dipl. ABT.

If you are interested in reading more about acupressure, I recommend this book as a great place to get started.

Before Getting Started: Massage Technique for Emotional Healing

For emotional healing, Gach recommends you massage your acupoints using your middle finger, supported by both the index and ring finger. You can also use your knuckles if that feels more comfortable.

He suggests you apply firm, steady pressure on each point, with your fingers held at a 90-degree angle. Then direct that pressure toward the center of the body. Gradually release that pressure toward the end of the practice, and end with twenty seconds of light touch for maximum effect. The length of time you hold this pressure will vary, but it generally ranges from two to four minutes.

To Head Off Anxiety

These first two poses are useful for easing symptoms of anxiety or warding off a panic attack.

Letting-Go Points

When you first feel the early-warning signs of an anxiety attack, Gach recommends finding the "letting-go" points, which are just below your collarbone (one on the left and one on the right). To find these points, begin by crossing your arms tightly over your chest, wrist over wrist. Chances are your fingertips will land on the spots we're talking about on your outer chest area, about three finger widths below your collarbone. I usually find this area is sore, but that may not be the case for you.

Once you've found each spot, Gach suggests holding the area firmly while you breathe deeply. I find massaging the area with a gentle circular motion works just as well. Try it both ways and see how it works for you. In addition to the deep belly breathing, I suggest repeating the word "relax" or "calm" to yourself.

If you're alone, you can say the word out loud, but repeating it mentally works just as well, in my experience. Or you can picture a white, calming light pouring through your body, relaxing you cell by cell. Again, give it a try and see what works best for you.

Repeat until calm.

Upholding Heaven

This pose is particularly useful for giving women an extra boost of confidence in situations where they might be tempted to back down. I recommend this pose for calming yourself before public speaking, tackling a difficult conversation, or taking on any challenge that requires a sense of focus and power you feel you might not have.

Stand in a relaxed pose, feet comfortably apart, arms loose by your sides. Inhale as you turn your palms up and slowly raise your arms overhead. Exhale as you interlace your fingers with your palms upward. Inhale again, pressing your arms upward, tilting your head back. Hold there a minute, allowing yourself to feel the power of the universe flow through you.

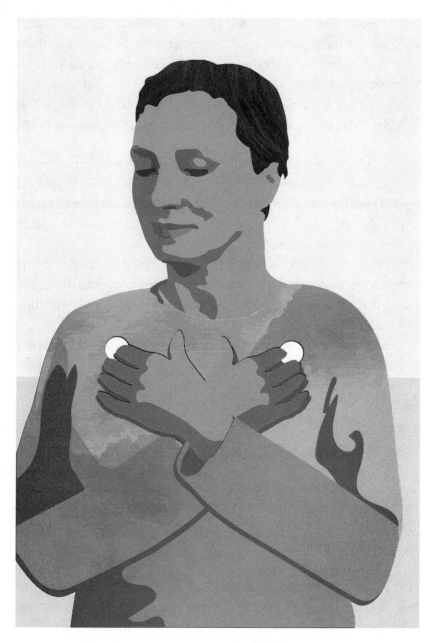

Letting-Go Points

At this point, I suggest you add some positive self-talk and/or visualization for added impact. If you want to try adding one of these options, you can focus on the words "success" or "I can do this," or whatever phrase makes you feel strong and capable. You may want to try a prayer, if that works for you. Or you can visualize yourself as Wonder Woman, standing confident and strong, cape flowing in the wind.

Now, imagine yourself being completely successful at whatever difficult task is before you. If you're going to speak in public, imagine yourself feeling fully confident in what you have to say. Picture everyone in the audience leaning forward; see them smiling and nodding as they enjoy your presentation.

If you're planning to have a tough conversation, imagine being surrounded by love and compassion as you share your thoughts. Imagine the person you're speaking with hearing you and answering in kind.

Once you have that image of success in mind, exhale as you lower your chin to your chest and allow your arms to float down to your sides. Repeat up to six times, each time feeling more confident and ready to take on the thing you fear. Repeat until calm.

For Use *While* Anxious: Waist Massage

Here's another great anxiety tamer. It's a simple, common pose you can use anywhere without anyone being the wiser—in line at the DMV, teaching your class, or standing in a restaurant waiting to meet your blind date.

Stand or sit in a relaxed pose. Put your hands on your waist, thumbs on your back, several inches apart. Now press firmly on one side of your body with your thumb and fingertips. Massage for two minutes as you allow yourself to breathe deeply into your fear. Then repeat on the other side.

As you continue to breathe deeply, you may want to visualize the stress and worry slowly melting away as the tension in your muscles

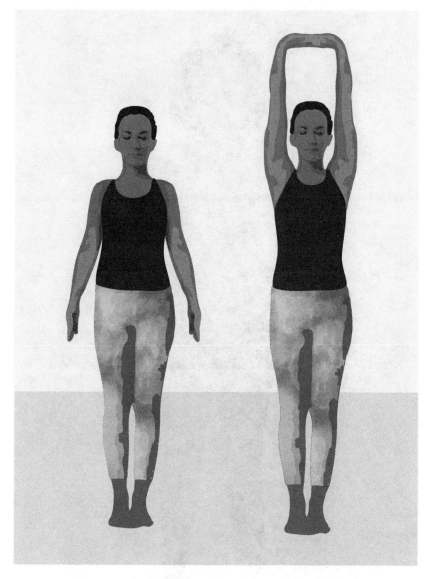

Upholding Heaven

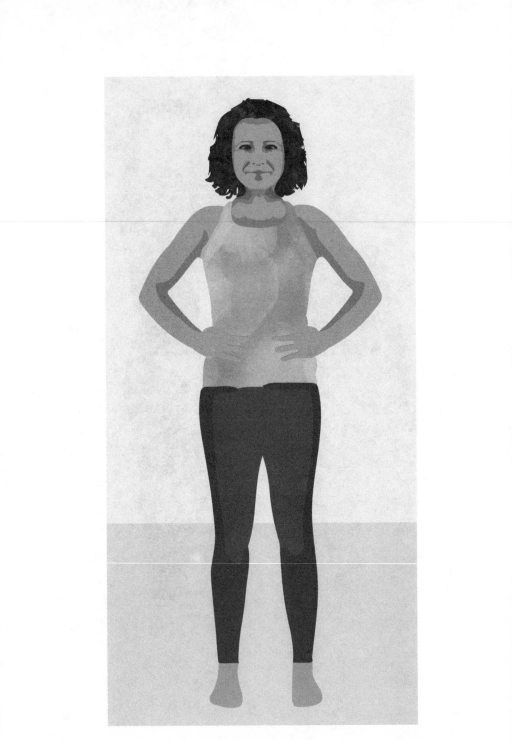

Waist Massage

238

eases and your breathing slows. You can also add a word/phrase of relaxation to repeat to yourself, for instance, "I breathe in peace. I breathe out fear." Repeat until calm.

For Use During a Panic Attack:
Sea of Tranquility

If you suffer from panic attacks, please give this one a try. It can be amazingly effective in easing your physical and emotional symptoms.

You'll find the Sea of Tranquility point located in the small indentation at the center of your breastbone. Take a minute to find it. Got it? Good. It often feels sore to the touch at first. But after a few moments of pressing or massage, that soreness will probably ease.

Once you've found the spot, press it gently while you breathe deeply, your belly soft. I find this point more effective for me if I massage the area with a gentle circular motion. So try both methods and do what works best.

As with the other exercises, you can focus on the word "calm" or "relax" as you breathe. (Feel free to pick a word or a phrase that resonates with you.) You might pray or visualize your body relaxing muscle by muscle, bone by bone, cell by cell. And as the tension flows out of your body, imagine a beautiful sense of calm flowing through you. Allow yourself to feel more peaceful with every breath you take. Do this for three minutes or until you feel calm.

To Increase Energy: Massaging Beside Kneecaps

I've used this point for years, especially on mornings after chemo for leukemia, when I was so tired I worried I wouldn't be able to get through the day. For me, it not only calmed my worries, but it also restored balance and energy to my body. I hope it will work the same way for you.

This point is located on your shinbone, about four finger widths below the outside of your kneecap. You can find it by cupping your

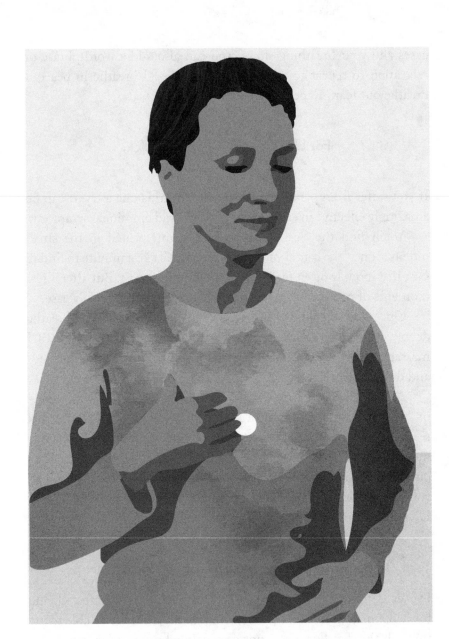

Sea of Tranquility

hands over the outside of your kneecap, fingers toward the floor. Once you do that, you'll probably find your fingertips are resting on the exact spot we're talking about. (You can make certain you've found the spot by keeping your heel on the ground as you flex your foot up and down a few times. If you're in the right place, you'll be able to feel your muscle tighten and release as you raise and lower your foot.)

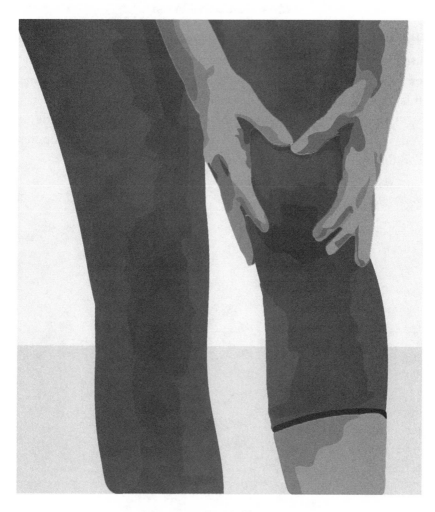

Massaging Beside Kneecaps

I've found massaging the spot in a gentle circular motion combined with some deep breathing also works really well. You may want to add some positive self-talk as you massage. You can also practice affirmations or visualize a renewed sense of energy and peace slowly filling your body. Repeat until calm.

To Relieve Anxiety and Nausea: Massaging the Wrist

This technique can be used to calm anxiety and can be particularly useful for dealing with morning sickness, nausea, monthly cramping, or anytime your stomach is upset. Best of all, research shows using this method is as effective as using drugs to treat the symptoms.

Using three fingers, simply press crosswise along the inside of your wrist where your watchband would sit. Hold for three minutes and then switch hands. Repeat until you feel calm.

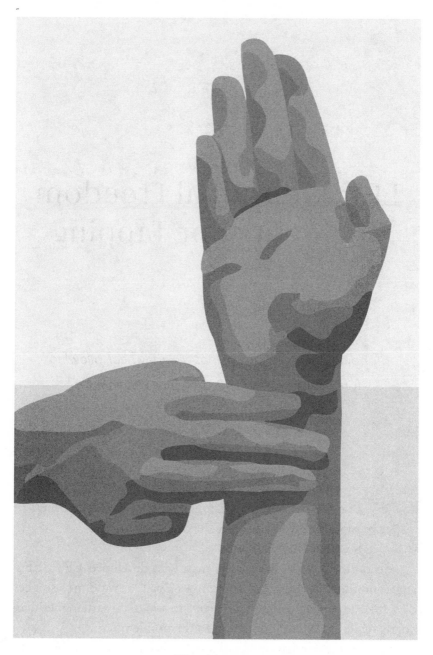

Wrist Massage

CHAPTER 42

EFT: Emotional Freedom Technique, or Tapping

Tapping is a powerful tool that can truly heal, allowing forgiveness, love, and acceptance into your life.

—Louise Hay, motivational speaker and author of
You Can Heal Your Life and *The Power Is Within You*

EFT IS often referred to as tapping and is one of the most effective tools for dealing with anxiety.

So, what is EFT?

According to Gary Craig, the man who developed EFT, "EFT is an emotional form of acupuncture except that we don't use needles. Instead, we tap with the fingertips to stimulate certain meridian points while the client is 'tuned in' to the problem."

Recent research has proven that EFT is effective in dealing with anxiety. In a study published in the *Journal of Nervous and Mental*

Disease, researchers found "the subjects using EFT showed significant improvements in anxiety as well as a significant decrease in cortisol [one of those stress hormones] level" after using EFT.

All right, you may be thinking, *we have proof it's effective. But how the heck does this tapping thing work?*

According to Craig, "Tapping on specific areas of the body opens the energy channels, or meridians, that run through our bodies and allows trapped, stagnant energy to flow freely."

Okay. What's a meridian? I like to think of the meridians in our bodies as highways and byways of the energy running through us. From time to time, shock, trauma, or just the stress of everyday life can block these systems, the same way red lights, stop signs, detours, and construction signs can stop the flow of traffic through a busy city.

Tapping on the ends of the meridians opens these blockages and allows the energy traffic to flow freely again. While tapping on its own can bring an instant sense of calm to the body, it's clear that the combination of testing, tapping, and talking brings the most relief.

Let's look at how this technique works so you can get a better idea of what I'm talking about.

EFT Technique

EFT involves the five Ts.

1. *Tune* in to what's bothering you. Really focus on your fears. Really feel the fear.
2. *Test* your level of your anxiety. (See the SUDS chart on p. 246.)
3. *Tap* along the end points of specific meridians to help release the energy blocks caused by fear, trauma, and negative thinking.

4. *Talk* as you tap about the things that are stressing you. Each time you tap a new place, repeat a focus phrase/word that works for you.

5. *Test* again when you've finished the tapping sequence to see if the process has worked for you. (See the SUDS chart.) If not, go right back to step 1 and begin again.

You can't do this wrong. Even though there are instructions and diagrams to guide you to where to tap, if you don't find the exact right spot, don't worry; you'll still get benefits from the process. Let me say it again: *You can't do this wrong*.

When to Tap

Anytime you feel anxious, consult the SUDS ratings scale to decide whether or not to use EFT to clear that anxiety. If your SUDS rating is lower than a 3 or 4, chances are what you're experiencing is a minor annoyance that will pass on its own. But if the rating is higher, chances are this anxiety is deeper and needs to be addressed.

Maybe this is an issue you've been dealing with for years. Maybe it's something new that just came up and is keeping you from living the life you want. Whatever it is, if your SUDS rating is above 4, doing EFT can help.

If you're not feeling particularly anxious at the moment and want to practice EFT, focus on something that will raise your anxiety to the 7 to 8 range. For instance: your boss, that funny sound in your

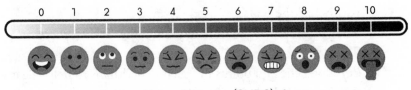

Subject Units of Distress (SUDS) chart

car, your unpaid student loans, the upcoming mammogram. You get the idea.

For example, Freida was terrified of spiders. Just the idea of seeing a spider made her shake and sweat. She rated her anxiety at 8–9 before she started tapping.

How and Where to Tap

Now that you're focused on something that makes you anxious, take a deep breath. Breathe deep into your belly. Let your shoulders go up in a shrug. Then, with a whoosh, let the air out and feel your body relax. (See "Shoulder or Shrug Breathing," p. 141.)

The EFT tapping sequence begins with what is called the karate chop. This involves tapping the outside edge of one hand (the part you would use to do a karate chop) against the flesh near the base knuckle of your index finger of the other hand.

Tap your hands together that way seven times as you repeat the phrase "Even though I'm afraid of heights [or spiders or whatever is on your mind], I love and approve of myself." If that phrase doesn't resonate with you, feel free to come up with a focus phrase that does.

Each time you tap a new place, repeat that focus phrase or focus word. For instance, you might repeat, "I feel my fear of heights lessening with each tap" or "I feel the stress in my body easing." You may find it easiest to just repeat the focus word "heights." The idea is to keep your focus on whatever is keeping you awake at night all the way through the tapping sequence.

Every time you repeat that focus phrase or word, notice the changing flow of energy. Is the tension in your body easing? Are your thoughts calming? Are you getting more or less anxious? Are you feeling more peaceful?

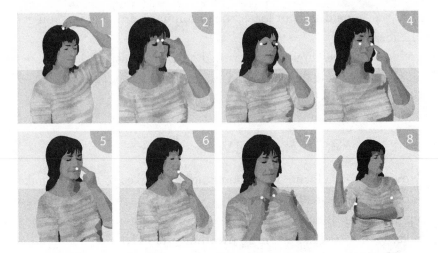

EFT Practice

Freida chose the phrase "Even though I'm afraid of spiders, I'm willing to let go of my fear" and repeated it each time she tapped in a new place. As she tapped, she noticed the tension in her shoulders softened and she started breathing more deeply. She also noticed that, for her, tapping under her nose seemed to be the most relaxing.

Now, all this may seem a little confusing at first, but don't worry. We're going to walk through it together step by step.

EFT Practice

1. With your index and middle fingers together, begin tapping on the crown of your head. Tap about seven times. (*A helpful hint*: Always start at the top of your body and work your way down.)

2. Now tap just above the bridge of your nose on the inside of your eyebrow, about seven times. (You can tap on either side, using either hand. If you like, you can use both hands and tap

on both sides of your body. Whatever feels best to you.) Be sure to remember that each time you move to a new tapping site, you're going to repeat your focus phrase.

3. Using the same technique, tap beside your eye at the outside corner while you repeat your focus phrase/word.

4. Then tap below your eye while you repeat your focus phrase/word.

5. Tap below your nose while you repeat your focus phrase/word.

6. Tap below your mouth while you repeat your focus phrase/word.

7. Tap in the hollow just below your collarbone while you repeat your focus phrase/word.

8. Finish by tapping under your arms while you repeat your phrase/word.

Once you've finished the complete series of tapping, stop. Take another deep, complete breath. It's time to reevaluate your anxiety.

Consult the SUDS rating scale to find where your anxiety is now. If your level has dropped to a comfortable 1 or 2, or if you're satisfied with how you feel, take another deep breath and get on with your day.

If your number is higher than you'd like, you can do another round of tapping. The good news is that you can do as many rounds of tapping as you need to feel peaceful again.

Freida didn't notice much change in her SUDS rating after the first few rounds of tapping. But by the fourth time through, she realized she was feeling much less anxious and was excited to find a technique she could use to finally help her face her fear.

You can tap as often as you like during the day. In fact, the more often you tap, the better you get at it and the calmer you feel.

If you try EFT and find it doesn't work for you, if you experience any unpleasant side effects, or if you just plain don't like it or don't want to do it, then *don't*.

If you like the idea of EFT but can't seem to make it work for you, you might want to try contacting a professional who has been trained in EFT and can help you get started.

CHAPTER 43

Heal with Water

Pure water is the world's first and foremost medicine.

—Slovakian proverb

WATER CALMS anxiety. Whether you drink it, bathe in it, or spend time relaxing beside it, water contains magical properties that soothe and heal your spirit, mind, and body. If you're interested in creating a calm, centered life, including water can make a real difference.

Drink It

One of the easiest ways to ease anxiety is to sip a glass of water. That may sound too simple to be true, but according to Amanda Carlson, RD, "Studies have shown that being just half a liter dehydrated can increase your cortisol levels . . . Staying in a good hydrated status can keep your stress levels down." In other words, drinking enough water throughout the day can help keep you calm.

So, how about you? How many glasses do you get in a day?

If you need to add a few more servings of H_2O a day, here are some great suggestions from Monica Nelson's article "How to Drink More Water Each Day."

1. Make it a habit to start every day with a big glass of water. It's easy to do, and beginning the day with such a positive step gets the morning off to a great start.
2. Include a glass of water before or after every meal. (This may also help you eat less, so if you're looking to lose weight, this could help with that as well.)
3. Flavor your water. You can add lemon, lime, cucumber, apple, citrus fruit, or even some fresh herbs to flavor the water and make it more interesting.
4. Make it bubbly. Adding bubbles to anything just increases the fun. Drinking sparkling water can make your day a little more festive, and what could be better than that?
5. Rethink the size of your glass.
    a. *Smaller*: If you're feeling daunted by having to get down eight ounces of water at once, opt for a smaller glass. Smaller servings can be easier to swallow and may make it easier to get in your eight by eight.
    b. *Larger*: On the other hand, if you find you're not getting in all your servings for the day, you may want to carry a larger water bottle with you.
6. Change the temperature.
    a. *Hot*: One way to sneak a serving of water into your morning routine is to start the day with a cup of hot water and lemon.
    b. *Cold*: If you prefer chilled water, you can always keep a pitcher of water in your refrigerator, then pour yourself a glass whenever the mood strikes.
    c. *Just right*: If cold water isn't your cup of tea (so to speak), try drinking your eight by eight at room temperature.

7. Keep your water handy. Lots of women carry water bottles with them these days. Good for them and good for you, too. Just seeing that water bottle may remind you to keep sipping throughout the day.

8. There's an app for that. Using an app like Waterlogged, MyFitnessPal, iDrated, or Daily Water can be an effective way to make sure you stay on target with your daily water consumption. For those of you who love spreadsheets and flowcharts, you can create your own system for keeping track. Finally, for anyone who prefers to go old-school, you can keep track in a journal or on a daily log.

You know the great old saying "An apple a day keeps the doctor away?" Well, here's a great new saying: "Eight glasses a day keeps anxiety away."

Go grab a glass of water, then come back and we'll talk some more about water.

Bathe in It

There's nothing like bathing to relax your muscles, soothe your frazzled nerves, and calm your spirit. Whether you prefer to soak in the tub or to take a quick shower, the daily ritual of washing with water does more than keep your body clean. It also brings a sense of calm and peace into your life. And it can be an important part of your plan to ease your anxiety.

Research appearing in the *Journal of Complementary Therapies in Medicine* found that soaking in warm water daily for eight weeks is more effective at easing anxiety than a prescription drug.

So if you're serious about creating peace in your life, schedule some time every day to bathe your body and soothe your spirit.

And the good news for pregnant women is that they can enjoy the comfort of a warm bath, too. As long as the water is no more than 98 degrees and you keep your soaking to ten minutes, a bath can be a great way to ease the pain in your lower back and any of the other aches that can be a part of pregnancy.

If you're interested in reading more about the comfort of bathing and comfort in general, I recommend *The Woman's Comfort Book* by Jennifer Louden.

Listen to It

Even the sound of water can soothe the spirit. The sound of the rain on the roof at night, the splash of a fountain, or the rhythmic rolling of the ocean waves all work like nature's music to comfort and restore. If you're interested in creating a soothing environment, consider adding a sound machine in your office or your bedroom (or any other room where you want to reduce stress). Tuning in to the sound of waves, rain, or a waterfall, ahhhhh . . .

Sit Beside It

Of course, actually spending time by a beautiful body of water, large or small, is also a wonderful way to ease stress and help you completely unwind. I have a friend who always heads for the beach when times get tough. Maybe you do, too.

As it says in the article "How Does Nature Impact Our Wellbeing?" written by Jean Larson and Mary Jo Kreitzer for the University of Minnesota's wellness website, "Exposure to nature not only makes you feel better emotionally, it contributes to your physical wellbeing, reducing blood pressure, heart rate, muscle tension, and the production of stress hormones."

Whether you spend an afternoon at a local beach, stroll beside a nearby pond, or take a break from shopping to watch a fountain splash and play, you're doing something great for yourself. Could you vacation near a beautiful stretch of water? How about going for a walk along the shore of a nearby lake? If you're looking to create a core of calm in your life, start right now to find ways to spend some time near water.

CHAPTER 44

Nourish Yourself

Food is the most widely abused anti-anxiety drug in America, and exercise is the most potent yet underutilized antidepressant.

—Bill Phillips, entrepreneur, speaker, publisher, and author of
Body for Life and *12 Weeks to Mental and Physical Strength*

I F YOU'RE like most women, you may be using to food to help ease your anxiety. Studies show that women are much more likely than men to turn to food when they're stressed. And 49 percent of us report having eaten too much or eaten unhealthy foods in the past month to help soothe our fears.

Me too. For years I coped with my anxiety by eating. Now, I'm not talking about snacking on an apple or enjoying salad at lunch. I'm talking about the embarrassing, out-of-control eating I hid from the world. Maybe you know what I'm talking about because you've done it yourself.

I'm talking about downing a half gallon of butter pecan ice cream, eating your way through a family-size pizza all by yourself, or polishing off the family-size bag of cheesy popcorn in one sitting (and then not remembering it—but knowing you did it because you have that sticky orange powder all over your hands). Yup—that's what I'm talking about when I say I used to use food to cope with my anxiety.

The problem was that I felt great while I was on the hunt for something to eat, and even better while I was munching those twelve chocolate chip cookies. Not a single anxious thought on the horizon. Just the fun of chewing and swallowing and some blessed moments of symptom-free peace. For me, eating piles of high-fat, salty, or sugary treats always worked—for a few minutes.

But the minute I put down the spoon, hid the empty bag at the bottom of the trash can, or washed my hands to get rid of the evidence, I would be more miserable than before I started eating.

I'd let myself down. And now I was not only anxious, but I was nauseated, guilty, and angry that I couldn't seem to get it through my head that food was only a temporary fix for my worry and fear.

Maybe you recognize yourself in that description. Maybe you know what it's like to promise you're going to stick to your healthy eating plan no matter what—starting tomorrow. And while you're making that promise to yourself, you call for Chinese takeout or rip open a package of Ho Hos because you're never going to eat those things again. Ever! This is positively, absolutely the last time you're going to binge eat. From now on you're going to live on celery and baked fish. You feel virtuous. You feel wonderful.

But tomorrow never seems to come.

Maybe you've been using food as a companion, as sedation or comfort late at night when you're alone with your fears. Maybe you've tried to deal with your overeating before, without success. Maybe you've just decided today that you're sick and tired of feeling sick and tired and are finally ready to do something about it.

No matter what your struggles with food look like, I strongly recommend the first step you take in healing your relationship with food is to start by asking your health care provider what approach to healthier eating would be best for you. Let her be your guide to making sure you're choosing the right food plan for you.

> If you've been diagnosed with an eating disorder, or if you think you may have an eating disorder, it's important to work with a professional as you move toward recovery.

The next step is to get some good support. You can enlist the help of friends and/or family. You can call a professional, join a group either in person or online, or enroll in a diet plan or program. But please be smart about the process. There are lots of books, diets, organizations, professionals, and websites out there that can offer you sound information on finding a sensible eating plan and support to help you stick with it. There are also lots of crazy fad diets that not only don't work, but they can actually harm your health.

Recovering from food issues (or any kind of addiction) can be a long, hard road, and I've found having company to guide and support you always makes the way easier.

In my own journey to healthy eating, I tried all sorts of things; some worked, some didn't. But I kept trying things until I found what worked for me. I suggest you do the same. Don't be afraid to try something new or to go back and try something again. Things change. You change.

In the end, what finally worked for me was changing my focus from using food to comfort or sedate myself to using food to nourish and heal my body. What a difference. For me, changing my focus meant I naturally began eating more fruits and vegetables. I ate protein at breakfast and gave up almost all refined sugar.

I also spent time getting in touch with my body, honoring it by listening to its signals. It was a revelation to me that I could count on my body to tell me when to eat and when to stop eating.

And I have learned that the secret to making that connection between body and mind is to slow the pace of eating until your brain and stomach have a chance to communicate (usually about twenty minutes).

If you're interested in learning to eat more slowly, here are some great techniques to get you started.

In-Touch Eating

Put your fork down from time to time. Take a breath. Take a break. Tune in to how your body is feeling. Say something witty to your dinner companion and then pick up your fork again. Try doing this once or twice during a meal, and if it works, gradually increase the number of eating breaks you take.

Focus on chewing your food. I assume you like food and enjoy the process of eating. Well, how often do you actually taste the food you're putting in your mouth? How often do you stop to enjoy the aroma? The texture? The flavor? How often have you eaten a meal without tasting a single bite? What do you think might happen if you started chewing your food thoroughly before shoveling in the next forkful?

Start listening for the sigh you make as you eat. A sigh? Really? You might not be aware (I know I wasn't), but that great, big sigh you make while you're eating is a clear signal that you're getting full. Once I started listening for that first sigh, I was shocked at how quickly I was sighing and how much I was eating afterward. I think of that sigh as the click you get when you're pumping gas, the one that means the tank is full and it's time to stop. When you sigh, you're full and it's time to stop.

Don't get too hungry! Don't skip meals, and be sure to include some healthy snacks every day. (Isn't it wonderful? We get to eat ourselves calm.) I now carry nuts and dried fruit with me to grab when I start getting that "hangry" (hungry/angry) feeling. Eating something when you're hungry (what a concept) makes good sense for both your body and your mood. That hunger is a signal that your body needs some fuel ASAP. Your blood sugar may be low, and low blood sugar can cause anxiety. Skipping meals, including breakfast, and/or going without food for long periods of time can actually contribute to your anxiety. No more starving. No more punishing yourself today for overeating yesterday. Promise yourself right here and now that you're going to listen to your body and feed it when it asks for food. (If you had a dog or a cat or a goldfish, I bet you'd feed it when it asked you for food, right? Why not treat yourself with the same kindness?)

Keep a food journal. Keeping track of what you actually eat can hold you accountable for what you're putting in your mouth. It gives you a record of what works for you and what doesn't and points out where and how you could make some changes. You can write everything down with pen and pencil or use an app like MyFitnessPal or SparkPeople. As always, do what works best for you.

It took me a while to make these new ways of eating a habit, but when I listened to my body, I ate less and felt better. I had a renewed feeling of energy, and a zest for life was a great incentive to keep at it. Now I can't imagine eating any other way. I still enjoy eating foods I love—they're just different foods. I still love thinking about food—I just think about it differently and I hope you will, too.

CHAPTER 45

Eat and Drink This

Good food is good mood.

—Author unknown

RESEARCH SHOWS that what we eat impacts not just how we feel physically, but how we feel *emotionally*. As Caroline Cassels writes in her article "Whole Diet May Ward Off Depression and Anxiety," "A traditional or whole diet characterized by vegetables, fruit, whole grains, and high-quality meat and fish may help prevent mental illness—specifically depression and anxiety."

That's pretty powerful information for any woman looking to create a calm, centered life. And if you want to eat in a way that soothes your anxiety and fuels your body in a healthy way, here are some tips to get you started.

How to Eat to Ease Anxiety

Daniel K. Hall-Flavin, MD, recommends the following rules for eating to cope with anxiety:

1. Start by eating a breakfast that includes protein. Protein keeps you full longer and keeps your blood sugar steady, which, in turn, keeps your mood steady. Include foods like eggs, peanut butter, cheese, or some yogurt in that first meal of the day.

2. Be sure to pay attention to food allergies. This one is important. Eating something you're sensitive to can make you miserable. If you think you're having a negative reaction to a particular food, keep a food journal for a week. That will help you narrow things down to what's really bothering you. Once you've identified the culprits, you can eliminate them from your diet. You might also want to talk to your health care provider about getting tested for allergies.

3. Do your best to eat balanced meals. Try to include something from all the food groups at every meal to help keep you satisfied longer and to keep your blood sugar steady. And the more color you can get on your plate, the healthier the meal. (M&M's and Skittles excluded. *You know what I mean.*)

What to Eat to Ease Anxiety

Now, here's some great news. There are a number of delicious foods we can eat to ease our worry, and they turn out to be things I bet you're already eating.

In her article "9 Foods That Help or Hurt Anxiety" in *Everyday Health*, Beth W. Orenstein recommends the following foods for stress relief:

Turkey. "Some researchers believe that tryptophan can have a positive effect on stress because this amino acid helps your brain produce feel-good chemicals."

You probably don't need any research to know that's true. You know how calm and relaxed you feel after eating a turkey dinner. So include foods like turkey, chicken, seafood, bananas, milk, oats, cheese, soy, nuts and seeds, eggs, and peanut butter in your diet for that calm "I've just eaten a turkey dinner" feeling.

Foods rich in vitamin B. "Studies have shown a relationship between the B vitamins, including thiamin or vitamin B_1, and mood. A deficiency in B vitamins, such as folic acid and B_{12}, can trigger depression in some people."

Foods that are high in the B vitamins include beef, pork, chicken, seafood, leafy greens, soy products, whole grains, milk, cheese, beans and peas, citrus fruits, nuts, and eggs.

Complex carbs. "Carbohydrates also increase production of serotonin in the brain." Lately carbs have gotten a bad reputation, but not all carbs are created equal. Complex carbohydrates can be an important part of a healthy diet. Healthy carbs include whole-grain breads, pastas, and cereals, barley, nuts and seeds, couscous, brown rice, quinoa, buckwheat, corn, and most fruits and vegetables.

Fish. "Studies have shown that patients who took omega-3 fatty acids along with their prescription antidepressants improved more than those who took antidepressants alone." Those servings of salmon, mackerel, anchovies, sardines, herring, fresh tuna, and lake trout that your cardiologist recommends to keep your heart healthy might also help lift your mood. So eat your fish.

Protein. "Protein helps stimulate the production of the brain chemicals norepinephrine and dopamine . . . Higher levels of norepinephrine and dopamine have been shown to improve alertness, mental energy, and reaction time." Including foods like Greek yogurt, fish, meats, cheese, eggs, nuts and seeds, beans and peas, and processed soy products in your meals and as snacks throughout your day can help give you the energy you need to get through the day, both physically and emotionally.

Dr Oz's Anti-Anxiety Elixir

If you're looking for a little something extra you can do to help you keep your calm, here's a great suggestion for an anti-anxiety elixir from Dr. Oz's Worry Cure & Diet Plan.

He recommends mixing together a teaspoon of lemon juice, a teaspoon of ground ginger, and a half teaspoon of honey. Stir the three ingredients together and take three times a day.

"Studies show that lemon juice lowers blood pressure by strengthening capillaries and may stimulate weak constitutions. Ginger calms the stomach, while honey controls the blood-sugar instability that accompanies worrying." Not only that, but it tastes delicious.

You can try the elixir exactly as written, or you can stir the lemon juice, ginger, and honey into a cup of hot water and then enjoy this elixir as a soothing cup of tea.

Herbal Tea

Drinking herbal or decaf tea can be a wonderful way to find a calm place in the middle of difficult circumstances. Aside from the medicinal qualities of some teas, sipping tea can be an excellent way to stay hydrated.

My two favorite teas for calming anxiety are chamomile and rooibos. And there's some research that shows why they work. As Dr. William Cole writes in his article on MindBodyGreen, "13 Foods to Help Ease Anxiety and Stress," "Chamomile tea has been shown to significantly decrease anxiety symptoms in just a few weeks," and rooibos tea "seems to work by having a balancing effect on the body's main stress hormone."

I know many women swear that peppermint tea helps ease their anxiety, and there is some suggestion that passionflower tea and lemon-balm tea can be useful as well. You may want to give them a try.

CHAPTER 46

Don't Eat or Drink This

If we're not willing to settle for junk living,
we certainly shouldn't settle for junk food.

—Sally Edwards, triathlete, speaker, and author of
Triathlons for Women and *Be a Better Runner*

Foods to Avoid

How and what you eat are not the only challenges when it comes to managing your anxiety in a healthy way. There are also some foods and drinks it's important to avoid.

Sugar

It may surprise you to learn that refined sugar (you know, the stuff you put in your coffee, you sprinkle on your cereal, and that shows up in most processed foods) can be a real problem for those of us who suffer from anxiety.

As Shelly Guillory writes in her article for Livestrong, "Foods That Trigger Anxiety," "After eating sugar, you may experience a short burst of energy, but then your blood-sugar levels drop, which can leave you feeling tired and sluggish. When blood-sugar levels get too low, known as hypoglycemia, you may experience symptoms of anxiety. When sugar levels swing from high to low, your hormones adrenaline and cortisol are released, which can cause anxiety and panic."

Caffeine

Another source of your anxiety may be that cup of coffee or tea you grab every morning to get yourself started. It wakes you up, keeps you up, makes you more alert, and can help you focus. But the surprising truth is that *caffeine is a drug* and it can also make you really anxious.

Is caffeine an issue for you? Let's find out. Take a minute and read over the list of symptoms.

Negative Effects of Caffeine on the Body

1. Anxiety
2. Irritability, crankiness
3. Difficulty concentrating
4. Thinking and/or talking faster
5. Insomnia
6. Digestive Issues (Acid reflux)
7. Rapid or uneven heartbeat
8. Headaches
9. Increased urination
10. Twitching, shakiness

If you suffer from even a couple of these symptoms, let's take a look at your caffeine consumption.

Here are some of the most common sources of caffeine:

- An eight-ounce cup of coffee has between 65 and 120 mgs of caffeine.
- An eight-ounce cup of decaf coffee has 2 to 4 mgs of caffeine.
- An eight-ounce cup of black tea can have between 20 and 110 mgs of caffeine, depending on brewing time.
- An eight-ounce cup of green tea has between 20 and 45 mgs. of caffeine.
- An 8.3-ounce serving of an energy drink has between 50 and 160 mgs of caffeine.
- An eight-ounce serving of hot chocolate has between 3 and 32 mgs of caffeine.
- A one-ounce serving of semisweet chocolate has 20 mgs of caffeine.

If you're taking any kind of medication, be sure to check the label for caffeine.

In general, guidelines recommend consuming not more than 400 mgs of caffeine a day. If you're taking in more than 400 mgs a day, or if you think caffeine is making you anxious or you're experiencing unpleasant symptoms, why not consider cutting back?

Here are some ways to make cutting back easier: Have one less cup of coffee in the morning or switch to decaf. Maybe you'd be willing to try drinking tea instead of coffee or replacing that energy drink with a glass of juice for an afternoon pick-me-up. How about substituting herbal or decaf tea in the evening? Not only could that be a delicious change of pace, but it may help you sleep more soundly. Win-win.

Would you be willing to brew your tea for a shorter time? How about choosing a piece of fruit in place of that ounce of chocolate?

IMPORTANT NOTE: No matter how you decide to cut back on your caffeine consumption, it's important to make changes gradually to avoid any of the unpleasant symptoms associated with caffeine withdrawal. Those symptoms can include headaches, fatigue or drowsiness, depression, crankiness, difficulty concentrating, anxiety, and flu-like symptoms.

Making one small change a week can be an effective way to ease up on all that caffeine without suffering, and that's what we're all about here.

CHAPTER 47

The Worry Box

Nerves and butterflies are fine—they're a physical sign that you're mentally ready and eager. You have to get the butterflies to fly in formation. That's the trick.

—Steve Bull, professional footballer and author of
The Game Plan and *The Return Journey*

WHEN I was going through chemo and was overwhelmed with anxiety, I found using a worry box was a really helpful way to ease my anxiety—one worry at a time. As I went through my day, I'd stop every now and then to ask myself, "What am I worried about right now?" Once I had an answer, I'd write it down as soon as possible. If that wasn't possible, I'd tuck that worry away in my memory to record later.

Each evening I'd spend a few minutes reading over the worries I had written down during the day and recording the ones I'd missed. Then I'd drop them all into my worry box. It sounds simple, but for me it was extremely powerful. It might be the same for you, if you're willing to give it a try.

If you're not interested in writing things down, you can use an app like the Worry Box, but I like having a physical worry box. Just seeing it reminds me that I don't have to let my worries ruin this moment. I can put them aside and fall asleep without any panicky thoughts to keep me awake.

If you're like me and want to go old-school, find a box or a container that works for you. I use an old decorative box, but you could use anything you have around the house that has a lid—an old sugar bowl, a cookie jar, a shoebox, or even a piggy bank with a slot big enough to drop a folded piece of paper through. You may have to experiment with a couple of containers until you find the one that's right for you. That's part of the adventure of self-discovery.

I did a few other things to make this tool work for me. First of all, I dated each worry as I wrote it out. Then I spent a moment or two thinking about how that worry made me feel both physically and emotionally. I focused on how hard that worry is on my body and all the negative thoughts that had created it. I didn't try to change those feelings. I just let myself *feel*.

Then I would pray briefly (you can always substitute a meditation, an affirmation, or any saying that resonates with you). Finally, I dropped the worry into the box, acknowledging the loving power of the Divine and turning that worry or fear over to that power.

Once I let go, I felt a sense of freedom, knowing I didn't have to carry those worries with me. I could put them aside for the time being. That's not to say I only had to put a worry into the box once to be done with it. There were some worries that went into the box over and over again. The more I used the worry box, the easier I found it to deal with the stresses of living through chemo and the concerns that followed treatment.

I kept my "worry slips" for a year and would take them out and read them from time to time. It was surprising to see how many of the things I'd worried about the most never happened! When I looked back, I realized those problems had all been resolved whether I worried about them or not.

Here was real proof that the only thing worry accomplishes is to make you miserable both physically and emotionally and to keep you from living an amazing, limitless life.

So drop your worries into your worry box and be ready for a newfound sense of calm and freedom.

CHAPTER 48

Journal

Journaling—Paying attention to the inside for the
purpose of living well from the outside.

—Lee Wise, outreach pastor, author, and blogger
for "Achieving Success on Purpose"

KYLA HAD kept a journal since her sixteenth birthday. She wrote in that journal every night because the act of writing helped her relax physically, and exploring her feelings on paper helped her get a new perspective on her own behavior and other people's reactions.

After her father's death, Kyla started writing letters to him in her journal. At first those letters were angry and full of pain at the way he'd treated her. But over time her feelings shifted and her anger eased. Writing those letters helped her look more closely at their difficult relationship and helped her deal with her feelings of loss, guilt, and grief.

As Kyla discovered, journaling daily can bring clarity and new insights into your worries. Journaling allows you to journey inward, to explore thoughts and emotions without judgment or criticism. Journaling can help you find that core of inner peace deep inside you.

According to Barbara Markway, PhD, "One of the most useful things you can do to combat stress and anxiety is to keep a running record of your thoughts on paper. There's simply no better way to learn about your thought processes than to write them down."

Getting Started

If you want to try journaling, start by assembling the right tools. Download a journal app, buy a paper journal, find a pen.

If you want to check in with your journal every night or every morning, put it beside your bed, where it can remind you to make an entry before you go to sleep or when you wake up. If you want to commit to writing two or three pages a day, mark them off in your journal in advance. Maybe you'd like to give yourself some kind of reward for being faithful about your writing. You can use gold stars, check marks, or little smiley faces. Whatever floats your boat.

Write every day, once a week, or whenever the spirit moves you. Maybe you want to write in purple ink or in crayon. Good for you.

The only rules here are the ones you make for yourself.

Techniques for Journaling

1. If you don't want to bother writing your thoughts, why not take a page (or a picture) from Instagram and tell your story in photos.
2. If you're using a paper journal, draw pictures of your life instead of writing about it. You don't have to be Rembrandt or Picasso to get your point across. Stick figures can be just as powerful as a detailed masterpiece, in exactly the same way that simple words work just as well as long, complicated words and complex sentences.

3. Scrapbooking is another way of recording and reviewing your life, and if it resonates with you, then do it.
4. Cut pictures out of magazines and paste them in your journal. Draw maps or diagrams of your day's adventures.

Make the Journal Your Own

Your entries can be long or short, with lots of detail or just plain facts. It's up to you. If you find yourself staring at a blank page or screen, wondering where to begin, why not start by writing about the day's weather. Describe the cold rain or the blue sky to get your fingers moving on the keyboard. Or you could recount the day's events as if you were reporting for the evening newscast. "I went to the grocery store. I went to work. My assistant was out sick. I came home. I ate spaghetti for dinner."

You'll find the writing gets easier as you connect to how you *feel* about going to work, going to the grocery store, and eating spaghetti. And that connection to your emotional reaction and your life in general is where you begin to see what is really going on underneath it all.

Switching Hands

One of the best ways I know to create that kind of dialogue on an even deeper level is a technique I call "switching hands."

Begin by writing any question you want answered with your dominant hand. (Righties use your right hand, lefties your left.) Then switch your pen to your other hand. Think a minute about that question, then write the answer to that question with your nondominant hand. Using your nondominant hand may feel a bit awkward, but using it to write your answers activates both sides of your brain in new ways. That can help create new connections and new ways of thinking.

Your writing will probably look like illegible scribble, but stick with it. Let the answer flow through your hand and onto your paper.

Give yourself all the time you need to get the answer on paper, and don't judge.

Once you've finished your answer, read it aloud. Are you surprised at what you've written? It's been my experience that the answer you get from using this technique comes straight from that profound, true sense of knowing deep inside you.

You can continue this dialogue with your inner self for as long as you like, and you can use it anytime you want to create a deeper conversation with yourself. I recommend it especially if you're feeling stuck or confused about something. Once again, do it only if it feels right for you.

CHAPTER 49

Plan to Worry

Never bear more than one trouble at a time. Some people
bear three kinds—all they have had, all they have now,
and all they expect to have.

—Edward Everett Hale, clergyman, historian, and author of
The Man Without a Country and *How to Do It*

S O WHY the heck do we worry? We're smart women. We
would never do anything we didn't think would make us feel
better. We wouldn't eat chocolate in the hopes of having bigger
butts (at least I wouldn't, and I bet you wouldn't, either). We eat
chocolate because we know from past experience it will make us feel
better in the moment. (It's how we feel *later* that's the problem.)

We don't worry because we want higher blood pressure, a nervous stomach, or insomnia. We worry because we believe something
positive will come from that worry. The question is, *What good do you*
expect to come from all your worrying?

I used to believe if I worried hard enough, nothing bad would
happen to me. I worried as practice for all sorts of terrifying situations.

I worried so I wouldn't be caught off guard. But no matter how hard I worried, bad things happened, and those bad things almost never turned out to be what I'd worried about. In fact, very few of my worries have actually happened—except in my imagination.

So, why do *you* worry?

"Are you kidding?" I bet you're saying back to me. "You think I'm worrying on *purpose*? I can't control my anxiety; it just happens. Believe me, *if I could stop worrying, I would.*"

I was an adult before I finally realized that lots of other women were living their lives without the fear or crippling self-doubt that was limiting my life. I was stunned and then curious. How the heck could I get to be like them? How could I be in charge of my anxiety, rather than the other way around?

It turns out, the answer is simple. *The way to take control of your anxiety is to schedule your worry.*

Let me explain.

According to Joe Brownstein's article "Planning 'Worry Time' May Help Ease Anxiety," researchers in the Netherlands found that "when people with adjustment disorders [a type of anxiety], burnout, or severe work problems used techniques to confine their worrying to a single, scheduled 30-minute period each day, they were better able to cope with their problems."

In other words, scheduling a time every day to worry helped women handle the challenges in their daily life more effectively. Now, that's good news. But here's even better news from that same study.

According to Thomas Borkovec, a professor emeritus of psychology at Penn State University, "When we're engaged in worry, it doesn't really help us for someone to tell us to stop worrying."

Interesting, but here's the real "aha" moment. He continues, "If you tell someone to postpone it [worry] for a while, they were able to actually do that."

To explore that idea, let's get back to the chocolate. Let's say Gwen's addicted to chocolate. She eats chocolate every day. She wishes she could stop eating so much chocolate, but she's tried to give it up a hundred times, with no success. She knows she can't give up chocolate!

And if someone told her that she was going to have to give up chocolate cold turkey, I bet she would probably panic and say, "I need that chocolate. It's an important part of my life, and *I am not giving it up*." Right?

But what if someone said, "Even if you're not ready to give up chocolate right now, would you be able to limit your chocolate consumption to once or twice a day?"

Do you feel the difference? Do you think it might be possible for Gwen to control her chocolate intake by enjoying a candy bar or two once or twice a day on a set schedule? Does that feel easier than giving it up entirely?

What about you? Do you think you could do it?

And if you could take that step to limit your chocolate, wouldn't you be in a much better place to take the next step to giving it up once and for all?

Well, planning your worry works the same way and can be an important first step in getting a handle on your anxiety.

By creating a schedule for worry, you can limit your "worry time" to an hour a day or less. Less worry means less wear and tear on your body. And if you're not worrying all day long, think of the time you'll have to enjoy yourself, think happy thoughts, or get stuff done.

Before we get started, let me caution you that this practice isn't for everyone. If you've experienced a trauma, are dealing with severe depression, or are feeling any discomfort during your worry time, discontinue it immediately and find a professional to guide you through your experience.

Scheduling Your Worry

Step One: Pick a place where you can worry without interruption. Then decide when and how long you're going to worry. Some women choose to worry for thirty minutes at a sitting, but you can worry for as little as ten minutes and still get good results.

Step Two: Anytime a worry shows up during the day, make a note of it. Remind yourself that you'll worry about it later. Then forget about it until your scheduled worry time.

Step Three: At your worry time, show up and worry.

Productive Ways to Worry "on Purpose"

There are lots of ways to worry, but we're looking for worry techniques that will help both to clarify your worries and to find ways to quiet your fears and your heart.

Here are some techniques to make sure you get the most out of your worry time:

Read the list of your worries out loud. Hearing those worries allows you to focus on them, brings order to your thoughts, and then helps you get in touch with the details of your anxiety.

Sit in front of a mirror and talk to yourself about what's worrying you. Talk to yourself like you're an old friend. Be honest. Don't judge yourself or what you're worried about. This is a time to really get to the core of what's making you so anxious.

Start with your biggest worry and tell yourself everything you know about it. Then take the worry and imagine it growing bigger and more terrible until it looks so ridiculous that you can laugh at it. You can do this visually, picturing your worry until it's huge and cartoon-like. Or you can exaggerate the story you tell yourself in the same way.

For instance, Joyce was worried about getting all her work done before the end of the month. She decided to try exaggerating her fears until they were as preposterous as she could make them.

She began by telling herself, "I'll never finish everything this month. This work is just overwhelming. I'll never be able to get it done. Everyone will be really angry at me. I'll get fired. I'll go broke. They'll take my car and I'll be homeless. They'll find me wandering in front of Tiffany's wearing nothing but a burlap bag and an old colander on my head . . ."

When she got to the colander, Joyce smiled and felt her whole body relax. By exaggerating her worries, she was able to take those worries less seriously. To her surprise, she found she was much less anxious about work.

Use your worries as a way to come up with solutions. Be creative, even silly about new ways to think about old problems. If you're having trouble with your best friend, you might imagine being stranded on a desert island with her and being forced to communicate.

What do you think you would talk about? What might you learn? The idea of being stranded might lead you to think that maybe a weekend away would help open new lines of communication. By using your worry time to look for answers, you may find things you've overlooked or come up with new, creative ways to deal with what's worrying you.

Record yourself worrying and play it back. Sometimes hearing or seeing yourself talking about your problems can be a real eye-opener. Remember, no judging, just open, honest communication with yourself.

Once you've finished worrying, imagine putting those worries away until your next worry session. Then get back to living your life with the sense of calm that comes from living your life without the constant hum of worry in your brain.

CHAPTER 50

Get Organized

Get rid of anything that isn't useful, beautiful, or joyful.

—Regina Brett, columnist, speaker, and author of
God Is Always Hiring and *God Never Blinks*

Organize

Zoey's house was a mess. Every morning she struggled to find her keys and her phone in the clutter as she headed out the door. And that made her consistently late. She'd almost stopped inviting friends to visit because it was so difficult to clean before they arrived, and she completely panicked when it came time to finding the paperwork to pay her taxes. She kept promising herself she was "going to get rid of all this stuff once and for all," but she was so overwhelmed she had no idea where to start.

How about you? Is your home clean and neatly organized, or is it packed with clutter and in need of a good spring cleaning? Do you have too much stuff? Is the stuff you *do* have neatly organized? Can you easily find the things you use every day? Do you know where your important papers are? Are your finances in order? Are you on top of your upcoming appointments, or do they sometimes catch you by surprise?

Do all your clothes fit? Are those clothes neatly stored, ready to be worn?

How about your refrigerator and pantry? Do you have nutritious, delicious foods on hand? Do you have cans in the back of your shelves that expired sometime in the last century? Do you have enough toilet paper and batteries to get you through the next week? Do your appliances all work? Is your purse neat and organized? Your wallet? What about your inbox and your desktop?

Does just reading these questions make you anxious? Maybe you're thinking that the clutter in your kitchen drawer or the mess in your basement has nothing to do with your anxiety, but I promise they do.

Every bit of clutter and every task you leave undone adds to the stress in your life. Being constantly surrounded by a mess can make you anxious and/or depressed. If you're living with mountains of laundry, piles of bills, and stacks of stuff, you're creating an atmosphere that allows worry and fear to flourish. And you're not alone.

In a survey done on behalf of HuffPost, 87 percent of the women surveyed reported anxiety over the state of their homes—that's almost nine out of ten of us.

So, if you're serious about creating a life of calm and ease, one of the most important things you can do is to start *now* to take charge of your environment. And if, like Zoey, you're feeling overwhelmed, here's a plan to get you started.

Get Some Help

On the day Zoey realized she was wearing a black shoe and a blue shoe in an important meeting with her clients, she decided she needed to do something about her life. She called her best friend, Natalie, an organization wiz, and they agreed to spend a Saturday bringing some peace and calm into Zoey's life.

Get Rid of Some Stuff

Zoey and Natalie decided to start by getting rid of the clutter—things like the one ski in the back of Zoey's coat closet, the jeans with the broken zipper, and the dried-up oil paints she hadn't used in eight years.

They began by making sure they had plenty of plastic bags to bag up the outgoing stuff. Then they focused on cleaning one room at a time, starting in the kitchen. There they went through her refrigerator, tossed out the vegetables that had started to look like failed science experiments, the expired condiments, and the moldy cheese. They got rid of an old set of dishes that she hated and had never used and a rolling pin.

As they went through the rest of the rooms they got rid of the following:

- Anything that was broken and not fixable
- Anything Zoey didn't like
- Anything she'd never used, including clothes with the tags on them
- Anything she thought someone else might like
- Anything she was tired of stepping over
- Anything covered with a thick layer of dust

They filled six bags with things that Zoey was happy to part with. Then they put the bags into Zoey's car so she could take two bags to the dumpster, drop two bags into the bin for donations at her grocery store, and bring two bags to the local women's shelter.

Put What's Important to You Where You Can Find It

Once the clutter was gone, they made a list of the things Zoey used every day and needed to be able to easily find. They put a basket for important papers on her kitchen countertop, where she was sure to see it. They put a hook by the door where Zoey could hang her keys and a large bin in the bottom of her closet for her boots, umbrella, and hiking shoes, where she was sure to see them as she reached for her coat.

They put like things together. Her gloves all went in the same basket. They lined up her purses together in her closet. Her shoes went on racks. Her hair products went in one drawer in the bathroom, her lotions in another, and her makeup in the third.

Once they'd gotten rid of some of the clutter and had a system for making daily living easier, they decided to get Zoey organized.

There's an App for That

They decided to organize Zoey's finances by using a money management app (like Quicken or Mint). That way she had all her information in one place and would know exactly where she stood with her spending.

Zoey also chose to use a scheduling app (like Cozi) to keep track of her appointments and her grocery list. No more promising to be in two places at once or forgetting to buy coffee creamer three weeks in a row.

The Payoff for Being Organized

After spending an entire Saturday getting her life on track, Zoey continued to clean out clutter and get her home in order. She was delighted to find that she felt less stressed in the morning, she was able to get to work on time, her shoes matched, and she enjoyed wearing some clothes she'd found in the back of her closet.

But she was surprised at some of the other benefits that came along with being organized. Once she got her finances in order, she realized she was overspending. She decided to cut back on her shopping and began to put away a little money every month. She also began entertaining more and enjoyed spending more time with her friends. And she followed her new rule faithfully: "Don't put anything down; put it away."

So how about you? Do you need to get rid of some clutter? Do you need to get organized in any part of your life? What would your life look like if you made some changes in your surroundings?

Getting Started

- Is there someone you could ask to help you get organized? Do you want to consider hiring a professional?
- What if you set aside a day or a weekend to put your life in order?
- I know several women who've made the commitment to get rid of one thing a day. Do you think that might work for you?
- Would it help you to make a graph or a chart of your progress?
- What if you imagined the good your old coat or shoes could do for someone else?
- What if by letting go of the old, you were allowing something new to flow into your life? Why not find out?

CHAPTER 51

Build a Great Support Team

You're the average of the five people
you spend the most time with.

—Jim Rohn, entrepreneur, speaker, and author of
The Art of Exceptional Living and *Leading an Inspired Life*

HAVING THE right people in your life can make the difference between succeeding or failing at creating and living a calm, centered life. Building a support team of people who are on a similar journey can help you get through the bad times and celebrate the good days.

If someone is a few steps ahead of you on the path, they can serve as a guide or a mentor to help you along the way. They can share their story and tips for success and may even show you a shortcut you might have missed. If you're a few steps ahead, you can take the opportunity to give back to those coming after you.

The People in Your Life

Let's take a few minutes to look at the people you spend the most time with. Write a list of the names here:

1.

2.

3.

   Now let's divide these people into three categories. In the first group, include people who have little or no impact on you emotionally. They may be professionals, coworkers, or even people who are pleasant, are useful, and you enjoy being with. They don't offer you much in the way of emotional support, but they don't criticize, judge, or give you heartburn, either. These are people you may want to continue to have in your life.

Write those names here and we'll begin building your very own support team.

People who might be a part of my support team:

1.

2.

3.

Now let's move on to the people who *don't* support you. You know who I'm talking about. The people you avoid at all costs. The ones who always have a negative comment or manage to make you feel like an incompetent moron. They can be family, friends, acquaintances, or people you work with.

No matter where they show up in your life, write them here.

People not ready to be a part of my support team:

1.

2.

3.

These people have what I've heard call PLOM disorder. PLOM stands for Poor Little Ol' Me, and I think it's one of the most contagious disorders known to mankind. If you sit next to someone with

PLOM disorder for just a few minutes, you'll feel yourself coming down with it. People with PLOM can make everyone around them miserable in a matter of minutes.

So, how to deal with the PLOM sufferers in your life? Here are some suggestions.

1. Have a conversation with them about how you could work together to create a more positive relationship.
2. Find ways to get together less often. You may also consider limiting the time you spend together. Explain to them that you'd be willing to get together from 2:00 to 3:30 p.m. on Saturday afternoon. Arrive at 2:00, and at 3:30 p.m. get up and leave.
3. Don't spend time alone with them. Including others in your interaction can help ease the tension and serve as a buffer between you and their negativity.
4. Finally, this person may be so toxic or difficult that you have no choice but to eliminate them from your life entirely. What actions would you need to take to let them go? If you're not sure, why not get some support to help you through the challenge of making this difficult change?

Enough of the negative. Let's look at the people you want on your team.

Assembling Your Team

Now, on to those wonderful people who support you. These are people you look forward to spending time with and who always make you feel better after you've been with them awhile.

Who supports you? Who lifts your spirits and makes you feel like you can do anything you put your mind to?

People who already are, or I'd like to have, on my support team:

1.

2.

3.

These amazing people are going to be the foundation of your support team. They're the people you're going to want to spend time with, learn from, and go to when you need a hand. Put a star next to their names, put their numbers on speed dial, and make a commitment to see as much of them as you can.

What if no one that positive comes to mind? Okay, this is the perfect time to expand your circle of friends. If you're on the hunt for positive people, join a group, club, or association of people with similar interests. Take a class, attend a seminar, step outside your comfort zone, and be ready to meet some new people.

Not everyone you meet is going to be upbeat or supportive, but if you're patient and persistent, you're going to find some people who are perfect for your support team.

How to Ask for Help

How you ask for help matters. Before you start telling someone your tale of woe about your first gray hair, the guy at work who keeps stealing your lunch from the refrigerator, or the thing with your insurance company, tell her that all you need from her is a listening ear and ask her to repeat at reasonable intervals throughout the story the phrase "You poor thing." That's it. She doesn't have to solve your problem, have an opinion about the problem, or even a point of view. Her job is just to repeat the chorus to your sad song until you feel better. Easy-peasy!

For an ongoing problem, you might consider joining a support group, either in person or online. (Again I urge some caution. Make sure you're dealing with a reputable website and give out personal info cautiously online.)

Hire a Professional

When creating a great support team, you might want to consider finding a mentor or hiring a coach to help you along the way. The nice thing about having a coach is they are always on your side. The coaching interaction is always focused on *your* best interest, and coaches have additional information and experience that friends and family might lack. A coach can offer insight and guidance that can often smooth the rough patches in the road you're traveling. And I've found a coach is a great resource to have on any team.

As you're looking to add to your support team, keep your eyes and heart open to the possibilities. The right person could turn up in the most unexpected way, and you don't want to miss them.

There are a number of other professionals you might want to hire to help you deal with your anxiety. If you're thinking of seeing a therapist, make sure you hire one that suits you. (See "How to Get Help," p. 52.) But there are lots of other people you can turn to who can help you feel better.

You may want to consult a nutritionist, hire a personal trainer, or see a Reiki professional or a hands-on healer. You might see a chiropractor, a meditation coach, a reflexologist, an acupuncturist, or a practitioner who specializes in EFT (see p. 244).

What professionals might be helpful for you? List them here:

1.

2.

3.

Let me end with my own version of one of my favorite stories about asking.

> A young girl was struggling to move a heavy rock out of the patch of ground where she and her mother were planting a garden. As her mother watched, the young girl tried lifting the rock, rolling it, and finally dragging it out of the way. But it was no use. The rock wouldn't budge. "I can't do it," she said to her mother.
>
> "Are you sure you've done everything possible?" her mother asked.
>
> "I'm sure," the young girl said impatiently. "There's nothing else I could have done."
>
> "You could have asked me," the mother answered with a smile.

CHAPTER 52

Do Good, Feel Better

If you want happiness for an hour, take a nap.
If you want happiness for a day, go fishing. If you want
happiness for a year, inherit a fortune. If you
want happiness for a lifetime, help somebody.

—Chinese proverb

I F YOU'RE feeling anxious and want to feel better instantly, find something nice to do for someone else—then do it. You don't have to make the kind of charitable donation that you hear about on the news. You don't have to cure cancer (although that would be great). You just have to do something that makes someone else's life better.

According to Mary Ann Christie Burnside's article "Intentional Acts of Kindness," published on Mindful.org, "Studies show that thinking about, observing or practicing a kind act stimulates the vagus nerve, which literally warms up the heart and may be closely connected to the brain's receptor networks for oxytocin, the soothing hormone involved in maternal bonding. Kindness also triggers the reward system in our brain's emotion regulation center releasing dopamine, the hormone that's associated with positive emotions and the sensation of a natural high."

In other words, the research shows *whether you witness, perform, or even think about a small act of kindness, you instantly feel better.*

Maybe you've experienced this "helper's high" yourself. Think back to a time when you helped a classmate with their homework, called a friend going through a tough time, or drove a coworker to work. Do you remember what it felt like to lend a hand?

Have you ever felt your heart fill with joy as you watched a news story about a Good Samaritan who pulled a baby from a burning car or rescued a drowning dog? How about the fun of watching people pitching in to build or renovate a house for someone in need?

As you remember those feelings, are you smiling? Can you feel the "feel-good hormones" flowing through you? The good news is that those warm, wonderful feelings are always available to you, no matter how anxious you are. If you give to someone else, you'll feel better. Doing something nice for someone else can also remind you that you have something important to offer this world. And the pleasure of giving lingers long after the gift is given. The memories of giving will re-create the same feelings of happiness in your body and your mind every time you revisit them.

All you have to do to reap the benefits of giving is to find someone in need and then fill that need. "Doing good" doesn't have to cost anything but a few minutes of your time and a little effort on your part. It doesn't have to be a long-term commitment (although it can be if you wish). You don't have to have a special talent or a big bank account. All you need is the willingness to help and to connect with someone who could use a hand. (Please *never* volunteer or give *anything* you cannot afford to give or aren't capable of doing. Only give from a place of abundance and love, not because you feel you have to. This is about giving freely and joyfully. Anything else will make you even more anxious.)

Donate

Maybe you're already giving, contributing, or volunteering in a way that's meaningful to you. If so, good for you—literally. But maybe you've just been talking about giving to that cause that's so close to your heart and haven't gotten around to it. If that's the case, this is a great time to go online, get out the checkbook, or tuck some cash in an envelope and mail it off.

While you fill out the form, write the check, or count out the bills, focus on the joy you feel in your heart. Be grateful that you have a little extra that you can give, and enjoy the wonderful feelings that follow.

Volunteer

If donating to charity isn't for you, there are lots of ways to give that don't involve money.

Is there someone close to you who could use a hand? If someone doesn't come to mind right away, you could always ask around. There are all sorts of needs that go unmet.

Does someone need a ride to a medical appointment? Is your friend having trouble with her son and need a sympathetic ear? Is your neighbor recovering from shoulder surgery and in need of someone to rake her lawn? Is this something you could realistically do?

Great. Do it.

Acts of Kindness

As you go through your day, look for people who could use a smile, a kind word, or a helping hand. It takes only a second to smile at the parents in a restaurant dealing with a crying baby or the harassed-looking clerk taking tickets at the local theater. Could you offer a kind word to the lonely-looking woman waiting for a bus?

Give a compliment. Look the other person in the eye and tell them that they matter. Write a thank-you note to the boss of that great waitress you had last week or write a great online review of that struggling new little shop. Let people know when they've done a good job. Say thank you as often as possible. Make people glad you came into their lives, then share in that wonderful connection that holds us all together.

Maybe you have a special talent that you could donate to help others. Maybe you're good at technology. There are countless senior citizens who could use a hand with their computers and would be thrilled to have your help.

Can you sing? Play the guitar? Dance? Act? There might be a hospital in your area that would love to have you spend time performing for their patients. Maybe you could contact the nursing homes, libraries, or schools in your area that could use that talent of yours to lift the hearts of others.

Audrey loves dogs. Every Saturday morning she volunteers at her local animal shelter by taking the dogs out for a walk. These dogs may not get a chance to get out at all during the rest of the week, so she's sure to show up for their weekly outing. She said the dogs "dance for joy" when they see her and that feeling stays with her throughout the week.

Can you type? Repair things? Cook? Bake? Speak another language? If you're housebound, how about making it a practice to send people birthday cards or uplifting emails or call people just to say "hi." There are lots of people who would love to hear from you—and what a lovely gift to be able to give.

We all have something to give. It's just a matter of fitting your special gifts with the needs around you. Please don't let your limitations limit your thinking or your giving.

Surprise people by giving. Imagine the fun of bringing everyone in the office hot coffee or ice cream. Think of the surprise of the person behind you on the turnpike if you pay their toll. (That happened to me once years ago, and I still remember the incredible feeling of joy at having someone give me such a wonderful unexpected gift.) Recently I heard about someone who left a message on the locker of every kid in a local middle school. When the kids got to school, every locker had a note on it that read, "You are beautiful." I'm still smiling as I imagine how those kids must have felt. As Maya Angelou said, "I have found that among its other benefits, giving liberates the soul of the giver. When you learn, teach. What you get, give."

Amen.

Create Your Own Anxiety-Free Day

Spend this day wisely, it's the only day you have.
You are younger today than you will ever be again.
Make use of it for the sake of tomorrow.

—Norman Cousins, professor, journalist, and author of
Anatomy of an Illness and *Human Options*

NOW LET'S look at how you can put these tools to work throughout your day to create a peaceful life. Remember, this is *your* day. Feel free to use any or all these techniques in the way that feels right for you.

Good Morning

Taking just a few minutes every morning for yourself can make a real difference in how your day goes. You don't have to do anything fancy or complicated. You don't even have to leave your bed to improve your mood for the whole day.

Before You Get Out of Bed

Use affirmations (see "DIY Affirmations," p. 109). What could be better than starting off your day with an uplifting message to yourself about the great day ahead? You can make up your own affirmation, or try one of the following:

- "I am so grateful to have a new day to enjoy."
- "Today I look forward to finding love and joy."
- "Today I look forward to unexpected surprises, miracles, and abundance."
- "Today I will keep peace and calm in my heart no matter what happens around me."
- "Today I know I will handle any challenge that lies ahead of me with ease and grace."

Visualize success (see "Visualization or Guided Imagery," p. 148). Imagine the day ahead going exactly the way you want it to. Imagine getting only green lights, having people do what they promise, eating delicious food, being on time, getting everything done on time, and feeling loved and supported everywhere you go and in everything that you do. Be bold and have fun with this. Picture yourself doing things easily, saying what you mean, dealing with things calmly, and feeling in control.

Ask yourself better questions (see "Ask Yourself Better Questions," p. 86). If you ask yourself a couple of empowering questions every morning, you'll find the valuable answers you get will automatically make your day better. For instance:

- "How many creative ways can I think of to tackle my work today?"

- "Who could I get to help me?"
- "How could I break it down into manageable steps?"
- "What am I going to look forward to today?"

My favorite blockbuster question is: "How can I make this day better?" I use it all day long, but it works really well in the morning to get the day off to a wonderful start.

Practice EFT (see "EFT," p. 244). If you've having anxious thoughts first thing in the morning, try starting your day with some tapping. You may not need to practice EFT every morning, but it can ease those Monday blues and calm the scary thoughts that make it hard to get out of bed. EFT is a great tool to use in the morning or anytime you're feeling panicky, worried, or overwhelmed.

Pray/meditate (see "Meditate," p. 146). Prayer and/or meditation can be a wonderful way to get a positive start to your day. You can use this quiet time before you get out of bed to remind yourself that you're never alone, that you're walking through life surrounded and guided by a powerful and loving spirit. You can also use this time to focus on finding that place of peace in your heart or to focus on any belief or idea that helps you feel a sense of calm.

Read something uplifting. Ida starts every morning by reading something that makes her heart sing and says that feeling often follows her into her day. If this sounds like something that might work for you, why not keep some inspiring reading material by your bed to reach for when you wake up?

Listen to something uplifting (see "Music," p. 191). What could be better than beginning your day by listening to some beautiful music? Why not keep your phone/radio close at hand, so you can enjoy some peaceful tunes in those first minutes of wakefulness? There are also loads of excellent inspirational talk videos, podcasts, and CDs you can use to help you start the day on the right foot, including my CD, *Creating a Calm Day*. Experiment to see what works for you.

Laugh (see "Laugh," p. 182). Last but not least, find something to make you laugh. Tell yourself a joke, remind yourself of the time you and your dog tumbled off the end of the dock, or recall that movie scene that still makes you laugh out loud. And if you can't make yourself laugh, see if you can make yourself smile. Then take that smile into your day.

Getting Out of Bed

Now that you're feeling great emotionally, let's get your body feeling great, too.

Begin by slowly stretching like a cat after its nap or by wiggling your fingers and toes to get your blood moving. Next, circle your ankles and wrists and feel the energy start to flow. Now raise your shoulders up to your ears and lower them again. As you continue to stretch and gently move your body, take a minute to be grateful for your body and all the ways it serves you throughout the day.

Once you feel fully awake mentally and physically, take your time and ease yourself out of bed.

Putting Your Body in Motion

Once you're on your feet, reach for the stars, then continue with an easy stretch like the Qigong posture "Opening the Curtains" (p. 229). Or you could just hang over like a rag doll, letting your head drop toward your knees, your arms swinging loosely. If you have time, try a few yoga poses (see "Yoga," p. 215) or do any kind of easy motion that brings life and energy into your joints and muscles.

If you're in a hurry, here's a quick way to jump-start your day.

Your Morning Quick-Start

1. Stand by your bed.
2. Rub your hands together until they warm up.
3. Massage your arms and upper legs briskly to get the blood and energy flowing.
4. Inhale deeply, then exhale with a big whoosh and repeat until you feel fully awake and energized.

Make This Day Count

As you head to the bathroom, imagine the incredible day you're about to experience. Then continue getting your morning off to a great start by drinking a big glass of water. (See "Drink It," p. 251.) Take a minute to look yourself in the eye in the mirror and tell yourself how much you love yourself and that the day ahead is going to be awesome. (Remember you don't have to believe your affirmations to have them work—you just have to say them as often as possible. So feel free to affirm big.)

If you've posted some affirmations in your bathroom, why not take a minute to read one or two aloud and repeat them to yourself as you step into the shower? Try the following:

- "I will move calmly and confidently through my day."
- "Today I will seek only good wherever I go."
- "Today I will be able to handle anything that happens to me— no matter what."
- "Today I will speak to myself kindly and encouragingly."

Next, sit down to a good breakfast. (All right, if you're in a hurry, grab a good breakfast—but make sure you eat.) Experts recommend you include some protein at breakfast to help you get through the morning without being hungry. I suggest you also include a serving of a fruit or a vegetable to make sure you get your quota for the day. (See "Eat and Drink This," p. 260.)

If you're sensitive to caffeine, you can sip a cup of herbal tea in place of your usual coffee or tea. (See "Caffeine," p. 265.) Or you could enjoy a serving of Dr. Oz's Anti-Anxiety Elixir (p. 263) to help soothe you into a peaceful morning.

If you're serious about getting your day off to a positive start, avoid listening to the news first thing in the morning. Take a quick peek at the weather report if you must, then get back to enjoying the peaceful thoughts about the day ahead.

If you commute by car or public transportation, you can use that time to listen to some music or read/listen to an uplifting book. Take the time to repeat an affirmation or two, or to imagine again how well things are going to go for you. Remember, every little moment you can focus on using your calm-techniques adds to creating a peaceful day.

Be Prepared

As you go through your day, carry with you a list of five or more of your favorite tools for creating calm in your life. You can keep that list on a note card or on any of your personal electronic devices. I bet you'll find just knowing you have such effective tools at hand will automatically lower your anxiety level.

To make sure you have all your bases covered, I suggest you include:

1. A technique to manage any emergency situation. For instance: CO_2 rebreathing (p. 144), EFT (p. 244), any acupressure point you find effective (p. 232), or a phrase that brings you instant calm.
2. At least one breathing technique (p. 139).
3. A way to manage your thinking. For instance: asking better questions (p. 86), reframing using CBT (cognitive behavioral therapy, p. 74) or letting go (p. 93).
4. A pose or a posture you can do to help you relax physically. For instance: the Standing Balance Pose (p. 217) or Arm Swinging (p. 228).
5. Finally, include a technique you haven't tried before but think might work for you.

Feel free to use these tools as often as necessary to get you through the day with a sense of ease and calm. The more you use them, the better you're going to feel.

Eat Well, Keep Moving

Keep your focus on eating and drinking wisely throughout the day. Make sure you drink enough water. It's important to stay hydrated. It's just as important to make sure you don't let yourself get too hungry. That means planning nutritious snacks to keep you going between meals. Tuck a whole-grain granola bar or a piece of fruit into your purse or knapsack on your way out the door.

No matter how busy you are, it's important to invest time in eating lunch—away from your desk, if possible. It may be tempting to work right through lunch, but you'll be calmer, smarter, and nicer all afternoon if you take a few minutes for yourself and get the right fuel in your body.

If you want to remain calm throughout the day, make sure you get up and move every few hours (every hour would be even better). You can do something as simple as standing up and sitting down ten times. You can touch your toes, do a few dance steps, or go for a walk. It doesn't really matter what you do. Just that you do it! (See "Get Moving," p. 200.)

If possible, take a short break midafternoon. Sip a cup of chamomile tea, do some deep breathing, enjoy a couple of funny YouTube videos, or better yet, go for a brisk ten-minute walk outside. You'll go back to work refreshed and more productive.

At the end of your day, enjoy a balanced, nutritious dinner and maybe take a short walk afterward. Then ease yourself into your peace-building evening routine.

Create a Peaceful End to Your Day

As we discussed in the section on sleep, there are a number of ways to create a calm environment as you transition from the challenges and chores of the day to a great night's sleep.

In addition to those suggestions, why not take a warm shower or bath to help you relax after your busy day (see "Bathe in It," p. 253)?

This is also a great time to record your worries in your journal (p. 271) or to drop those worries into your worry box (p. 268).

Although you're probably not going to want to do any strenuous exercise this late in the day, try a few easy qigong moves (p. 224) or some gentle yoga poses like the restorative Legs Up the Wall Pose (p. 219) to calm yourself.

Another technique you can use to reinforce all the positive things that happened during your day is to ask yourself some questions that help you focus on the good.

All right, I hear you. You had a day when absolutely nothing went right! Nothing!!!

Well, let me challenge that a little. I bet there were *some* good things along the way. It's just that you're going to have to dig a little deeper than usual to find them. Did you have a great meal? Did you have an interesting conversation? Did you hear some good music? Did you see something beautiful? Did you do something for someone else? Did someone help you?

I know that even on your worst day ever, there was something positive that you could focus on for a few minutes before bed. Allowing yourself to acknowledge the good opens the door for more good to flow to you.

Other questions you can ask yourself might be:

- "What tools did I use today?"
- "Did they work?"
- "What other tools could I have used?"
- "What am I looking forward to tomorrow?"
- "What worries do I need to let go of, put aside, or drop into my worry box now, so I can have worry-free sleep tonight?"
- "What does my body need now to relax more fully?"
- "What's one thing I could do to bring a sense of peace into my life right now?"
- "What thoughts would help me ease into a good night's sleep?"
- "What am I looking forward to tomorrow?"

Or you might want to try some affirmations:

- "I can't wait to see what magic and miracles await me in the morning."
- "I enjoy doing everything I can to make sure I will fall easily into a deep sleep."
- "I let go of today's troubles and allow the peace and quiet of the night to surround me and keep me safe."
- "My heart is at peace. My mind is at peace. My body is at peace. I am at peace."
- "I exhale the cares of my day. I inhale the healing stillness of the evening."
- "I now allow myself to drift into a restful sleep and know I will wake refreshed and ready for tomorrow."

If you find you have trouble falling asleep or you wake up in the middle of the night, you can use the qigong technique Overwhelmed, Lying Down/Middle of the Night (p. 230) or the Corpse Pose (p. 222) to help you relax into a peaceful night's rest.

So that's what a day looks like using the tools and techniques we've been talking about. You can use them as written. You can use one or two together for a more powerful technique, you can just do part of a technique, or you can reshape the technique until it's just right for you.

Carpe diem.

Author's Note:
The Journey Ahead

End your day by privately looking directly into your eyes in the mirror and saying "I love you." Do this for thirty days and watch how you transform.

—Mark Victor Hansen, motivational speaker and author of the Chicken Soup for the Soul series

LIVING A life of calm and joy isn't some airy-fairy idea. It's something you create by taking persistent, consistent steps toward that goal every day. It's about forgiving yourself for your mistakes, your past, and everything else you've been yelling at yourself about over the years.

It's about having a plan in place for the tough days and reminding yourself to celebrate the good days. It's about putting yourself first, loving yourself, and, most of all, believing that you deserve and will have the calm, joy-filled life of your dreams.

And now that you have the tools, the support, and the plan to make your dreams come true, it's time to go out and create the life you were born to live.

As you open your arms and your heart to the adventures ahead, please know you're not alone. When you have a tough day, come on back here and read the passages that inspire you. When you're anxious, come back and try a new technique or reread a passage that helped you last time.

Please remember you are never alone.

So let's end as we began. Together. Traveling companions on the road to our own best life.

It has been my joy to travel this road with you, my friend, and I wish you well in the journey ahead.

Warmly,
Wendy

Additional Resources

The Anxious Brain

Brizendine, Louann, MD. 2006. *The Female Brain*. New York: Morgan Road Books.

Sax, Leonard. 2005. *Why Gender Matters: What Parents and Teachers Need to Know About the Emerging Science of Sex Differences*. New York: Doubleday.

What I Think Is Making Me Anxious

Ellis, Albert, PhD, and Robert A. Harper, PhD. 1991. *A Guide to Rational Living*. Woodland Hill, California: Wilshire Book Company.

————.1998. *How to Control Your Anxiety Before It Controls You*. New York: Kensington Publishing Company.

How I Think Is Making Me Anxious, Too

Burns, David D. 1999. *Feeling Good: The New Mood Therapy*. New York: HarperCollins.

————. 1999. *The Feeling Good Handbook*. New York: Penguin Putnam, Inc.

Reframing

Bandler, Richard, and John Grinder. 1982. *Reframing: Neuro-Linguistic Programming and the Transformation of Meaning*. Moab, Utah: Real People Press.

Robbins, Tony. 1986. *Unlimited Power: The Science of Personal Power*. Chapter XVI, "Reframing: The Power of Perspective," 289–313. New York: Simon & Schuster.

A Reframe of Reframing
Katie, Byron, and Stephen Mitchell. 2002. *Loving What Is: Four Questions That Can Change Your Life*. New York: Harmony Books.

Ask Yourself Better Questions
Robbins, Tony. 1991. *Awaken the Giant Within: How to Take Immediate Control of Your Mental, Emotional, Physical, and Financial Destiny*. New York: Simon & Schuster.

Let Go
Dwoskin, Hale. 2007. *The Sedona Method: Your Key to Lasting Success, Peace, and Emotional Well-Being*. Sedona: Sedona Press.

Gawain, Shakti. 1978. *Creative Visualization*. Mill Valley, California: Bantam Books.

Face Your Fears
Jeffers, Susan. 1987. *Feel the Fear and Do It Anyway*. New York: Random House Publishing.

———. 1996. *End the Struggle and Dance with Life*. New York: St. Martin's Press.

———.1998. *Feel the Fear . . . and Beyond*. New York: Random House Publishing.

———. 2003. *Embracing Uncertainty*. New York: St. Martin's Press.

DIY Affirmations
Hay, Louise. 1987. *You Can Heal Your Life*. Santa Monica: Hay House.

———. 1991. *The Power Is Within You*. Santa Monica: Hay House.

Just Do One Small Thing
Maruer, Robert, PhD. 2004. *One Small Step Can Change Your Life: The Kaizen Way*. New York: Workman Publishing Company.

Gratitude
Ban Breathnach, Sarah. 2009. *Simple Abundance: A Daybook of Comfort and Joy*. New York: Grand Central Publishing.

Just Breathe

Gordon, James S., MD. 2008. *Unstuck: Your Guide to the Seven-Stage Journey Out of Depression.* New York: Penguin Group.

Brown, Richard P., MD., and Patricia L. Gerbarg, MD. 2012. *The Healing Power of the Breath: Simple Techniques to Reduce Stress and Anxiety, Enhance Concentration, and Balance Your Emotions.* Boston: Shambhala Publications, Inc.

Meditate

Hay, Louise. 1988. *Morning and Evening Meditations* (CD).

Leeds, Wendy. 2017. *Creating a Calm Day: Your Daily Guide to a Peaceful Meditative Life* (CD).

Just Say No

Richardson, Cheryl. 1999. *Take Time for Your Life: A 7-Step Program for Creating the Life You Want.* New York: Random House Publishing.

———. 2002. *Stand Up for Your Life: A Practical Step-by-Step Plan to Build Inner Confidence and Personal Power.* New York: Simon and Schuster.

Anchoring

Bandler, R., and J. Grinder. 1975. *The Structure of Magic: A Book About Language and Therapy.* Palo Alto, California: Science and Behavior Books.

Robbins, Tony. 1986. *Unlimited Power: The Science of Personal Power.* New York: Simon & Schuster, Inc.

Play

Hoehn, Charlie. 2014. *Play It Away: A Workaholic's Cure for Anxiety.* Self-published.

Get Moving

Otto, Michael, and Jasper A. Smits. 2011. *Exercise for Mood and Anxiety: Proven Strategies for Overcoming Depression and Enhancing Well-Being.* New York: Oxford University Press.

Keep Moving, Stay Motivated
Duhigg, Charles. 2012. *The Power of Habit: Why We Do What We Do in Life and Business.* New York: Random House Publishing.

Yoga
McCall, Timothy, MD. 2007. *Yoga as Medicine: The Yogic Prescription for Health and Healing.* New York: Bantam Dell.

Qigong
Lam, Kam Chuen. 2014. *The Qigong Workbook for Anxiety: Powerful Energy Practices to Rebalance Your Nervous System and Free Yourself from Fear.* Oakland: New Harbinger Publications, Inc.

Acupressure
Gach, Michael Reed, PhD, and Beth Ann Henning. 2004. *Acupressure for Emotional Healing.* New York: Bantam Dell.

EFT: Emotional Freedom Technique, or Tapping
Craig, Gary. 2008. *The EFT Manual.* Santa Rosa, California: Energy Psychology Press.
Mountrose, Phillip, and Jane Mountrose. 2006. *The Heart & Soul of EFT and Beyond: A Soulful Exploration of the Emotional Freedom Techniques and Holistic Healing.* Arroyo Grande, California: Holistic Communications.

Heal with Water
Louden, Jennifer. 2004. *The Woman's Comfort Book: A Self-Nurturing Guide for Restoring Balance in Your Life.* New York: HarperCollins.

Bibliography

Introduction

P. xv
"Women in this country are twice as likely to be diagnosed . . ."
Compiled by Anxiety and Depression Association of America. 2016. "Girls and Women: Facts." Anxiety and Depression Association of America. Retrieved from: https://adaa.org/living-with-anxiety/women/facts

P. xv
"One out of four American women is prescribed medication . . ."
Bindley, Katherine. November 16, 2011. "Women and Prescription Drugs: One in Four Takes Mental Health Meds." Huffington Post.
Retrieved from: https://www.huffpost.com/entry/women-and-prescription-drug-use_n1098023

Part One: Name Your Anxiety

The Anxious Brain

P. 3
"As Regina Bailey explains in her article 'Amygdala's Location and Function' . . ."
Bailey, Regina. November 16, 2017. "Amygdala's Location and Function. Fear and the Amygdala." ThoughtCo. Retrieved from: https://www.thoughtco.com/amygdala-anatomy-373211

P. 6
"Now, it's important to remember we're talking in generalities here . . ."
Jantz, Gregory L., PhD. February 27, 2014. "Brain Differences Between Genders." *Psychology Today*. Retrieved from: https://www.psychologytoday.com/us/blog/hope-relationships/201402/brain-differences-between-genders

P. 6
"For years we believed that the human reaction to stress was . . ."
Brizendine, Louann, MD. 2006. *The Female Brain*. New York: Morgan Road Books, page 42.

P. 7
"But in female brains, that circuit of aggression is more connected to . . ."
Brizendine, Louann, MD. 2006. *The Female Brain*. New York: Morgan Road Books, page 42.

P. 7
"When I'm stressed, all I want to do is avoid human contact. And I've . . ."
Sax, Leonard. 2005. *Why Gender Matters: What Parents and Teachers Need to Know About the Emerging Science of Sex Differences*. New York: Doubleday, page 29.

P. 7
"Research shows that in women, there tends to be more blood flow . . ."
Jantz, Gregory L., PhD. February 27, 2014. "Brain Differences Between Genders." *Psychology Today*. Retrieved from: https://www.psychologytoday.com/us/blog/hope-relationships/201402/brain-differences-between-genders

P. 7
"Women are more likely to remember and rethink the past in greater detail . . ."
Brizendine, Louann, MD. 2006. *The Female Brain*. New York: Morgan Road Books, page 127.

P. 8
"Memories in men tend to be short and sweet . . ."

Brizendine, Louann, MD. 2006. *The Female Brain*. New York: Morgan Road Books, page 127.

P. 8
"We know that anxiety looks different in our brains . . . Brain scans show us . . ."
Nield, David. August 9, 2017. "Women's Brains Have More Blood Flow Than Men's, New Study Shows," *Science Alert*. Retrieved from: https://www.sciencealert.com/women-s-brains-are-more-active-than -men-s-shows-a-new-study

P. 8
"Over the course of their lifetime, women are 60 percent more likely . . ."
Castillo, Michelle. June 7, 2012. "Anxiety Causes Women's Brains to Work Harder Than Men's." *CBS News*. Retrieved from: https://www.cbsnews. com/news/anxiety-causes-womens-brains-to-work-harder-than-mens/

Why Women Worry

P. 12
"But in the last few years, researchers have located a specific gene . . ."
Bergland, Christopher. March 11, 2017. "Genetics Play a Role in Social Anxiety Disorder, Study Finds." *Psychology Today*. Retrieved from: https://www.psychologytoday.com/us/blog/the-athletes-way/201703/ genetics-play-role-in-social-anxiety-disorder-study-finds

P. 12
". . . a gene that is considered a factor in developing panic disorder."
Centre for Genomic Regulation. November 28, 2013. "Gene Found Responsible for Susceptibility to Panic Disorder." *Science Daily*. Retrieved from: https://www.sciencedaily.com/releases/2013/11/131128133921.htm

P. 12
"Research has also found that there's a tendency for generalized anxiety . . ."
Lucia, Jonathan. 2004. "Generalized Anxiety Disorder." *Appalachian State University*.

P. 12
"According to Olivia Remes, one of the reasons women are . . ."
Remes, Olivia. June 10, 2016. "Women Are Far More Anxious than Men—Here's the Science." *The Conversation*. Retrieved from: https://the conversation.com/women-are-far-more-anxious-than-men-heres-the -science-60458

P. 13
"As Joel Young writes in *Psychology Today* . . ."
Young, Joel, MD. April 22, 2015. "Women and Mental Illness." *Psychology Today*. Retrieved from: https://www.psychologytoday.com/blog/when-your-adult -child-breaks-your-heart/201504/women-and-mental-illness

P. 13
"It's no wonder we're so anxious . . ."
Edited by Talkspace. February 2, 2017. "Anxiety Symptoms in Women: A Quick Guide." *Talkspace*. Retrieved from: https://www.talkspace.com/ blog/2017/02/anxiety-symptoms-in-women-quick-guide/

P. 13
"It's no wonder we're *three times* more likely to be diagnosed with PTSD . . ."
Vogt, Dawne, PhD. February 23, 2016. "Research on Women, Trauma and PTSD." U.S. Department of Veterans Affairs. Retrieved from: https:// www.ptsd.va.gov/professional/treat/specific/ptsd_research_women.asp

P. 13
"As Michael J. Mufson, MD, a Harvard psychiatrist, writes . . ."
Mufson, Michael J., MD. 2017. "Can a Traumatic Event Cause Anxiety Disorders?" Sharecare. Retrieved from: https://www.sharecare .com/health/anxiety-disorder-causes-and-risk-factorscan-traumatic -event-anxiety-disorders

P. 15
"Taylor Clark suggests in her article in *Slate* that . . ."
Clark, Taylor. April 20, 2011. "Nervous Nellies." *Slate*. Retrieved from: http://www.slate.com/articles/life/family/2011/04/nervous_nellies.html

P. 15
"If Mary hangs back shyly from joining the other children . . ."
Davenport, Barrie. October 26, 2015. "24 Anxiety Symptoms in Women and How to Annihilate Them." *Live Bold and Bloom*. Retrieved from: https://liveboldandbloom.com/10/health/anxiety-symptoms-in-women

P. 15
"What happens if Mary gets stuck halfway up . . ."
Clark, Taylor. April 20, 2011. "Nervous Nellies." *Slate*. Retrieved from: http://www.slate.com/articles/life/family/2011/04/nervous_nellies.html

P. 17
"We have to work harder to get the credit we deserve . . ."
Young, Joel, MD. April 22, 2015. "Women and Mental Illness." *Psychology Today*. Retrieved from: https://www.psychologytoday.com/blog/when-your-adult-child-breaks-your-heart/201504/women-and-mental-illness

P. 17
"Women are much more likely to lose sleep worrying . . ."
Kossman, Sienna. April 21, 2016. "Poll: Women Lose More Sleep Over Money Worries than Men." *CreditCards.com*. Retrieved from: https://www.creditcards.com/credit-card-news/poll-women-more-sleepless-nights.php

P. 17
We're also more likely to live in poverty . . ."
Davenport, Barrie. October 26, 2015. "24 Anxiety Symptoms in Women and How to Annihilate Them." *Live Bold and Bloom*. Retrieved from: https://liveboldandbloom.com/10/health/anxiety-symptoms-in-women

P. 17
"Women are still paid only three-quarters of what men are paid for the same job . . ."
Mellan, Olivia, and Karina Piskaldo. Reviewed June 9, 2016. "Men, Women, and Money." *Psychology Today*. Retrieved from: https://www.psychologytoday.com/articles/199901/men-women-and-money

P. 17
"We're the ones who take time off to care for children . . ."
Chatzky, Jean. September 29, 2017. "Putting Finance in Perspective." Jackson.com.

P. 17
"To add insult to injury, we're likely to live seven years longer than men . . ."
Mellan, Olivia, and Karina Piskaldo. Reviewed June 9, 2016. "Men, Women, and Money." *Psychology Today*. Retrieved from: https://www.psychologytoday.com/articles/199901/men-women-and-money

P. 17
"When a major financial institution asked high school students . . ."
Mellan, Olivia, and Karina Piskaldo. Reviewed June 9, 2016. "Men, Women, and Money." *Psychology Today*. Retrieved from: https://www.psychologytoday.com/articles/199901/men-women-and-money

P. 18
"Studies show that it's much more important for women to have good relationships . . ."
Edited by the American Psychological Association. 2017. "Gender and Stress." American Psychological Association. Retrieved from: http://www.apa.org/news/press/releases/stress/2010/gender-stress.aspx

P. 18
"We're the ones who are more likely to worry about the health of our partners . . ."
Edited by ABC News. February 23, 2006. "Do Men or Women Worry More?" *ABC News*. Retrieved from: http://abcnews.go.com/GMA/Health/story?id=1653218

P. 18
"We run ourselves ragged trying to balance . . ."
Edited by Talkspace. February 2, 2017. "Anxiety Symptoms in Women: A Quick Guide." *Talkspace*. Retrieved from: https://www.talkspace.com/blog/2017/02/anxiety-symptoms-in-women-quick-guide/

P. 19
"According to a survey done by the Pew Research Center . . ."
Andrews, Linda Wasmer. June 9, 2015. "Why Women Need More Me-Time—and How They Can Claim It." *Psychology Today*. Retrieved from: https://www.psychologytoday.com/blog/minding-the-body/201506/why-women-need-more-me-time-and-how-they-can-claim-it

P. 19
"And according to a study conducted by *Real Simple* and the Families and Work . . ."
Edited by Real Simple. April 4, 2012. "How Do Women Spend Their Time?" *Real Simple*. Retrieved from: https://www.realsimple.com/work-life/life-strategies/time-management/spend-time#illo-melting-hourglass

The Price We Pay for Being Anxious

P. 29
"To her surprise, the doctor told her her headaches could be a symptom . . ."
Edited by Harvard Medical School. Updated May 9, 2018. "Anxiety and Physical Illness." Harvard Health Publishing. Retrieved from: https://www.health.harvard.edu/staying-healthy/anxiety_and_physical_illness

A Checklist of Your Anxiety Symptoms

P. 34
"A majority of women report having physical symptoms of anxiety . . ."
Edited by the American Psychological Association. 2017. "Gender and Stress." American Psychological Association. Retrieved from: http://www.apa.org/news/press/releases/stress/2010/gender-stress.aspx

Where to Start

P. 35
"In *Yoga as Medicine*, Timothy McCall describes a study done . . ."
McCall, Timothy, MD. 2007. *Yoga as Medicine*. New York: Bantam Dell, pages 138–139.

P. 35
"As Kabat-Zinn says, 'People need different doors . . .'"
McCall, Timothy, MD. 2007. *Yoga as Medicine*. New York: Bantam Dell, page 139.

When to Get Help

P. 51
"David Sack, MD, reports in a study published . . ."
Sack, David, MD. March 18, 2013. "5 Signs It's Time to Seek Therapy." *Psychology Today*. Retrieved from: https://www.psychologytoday.com/blog/where-science-meets-the-steps/201303/5-signs-its-time-seek-therapy

How to Get Help

P. 52
"According to an article in *Consumer Reports*, studies show that 'people who . . .'"
Edited by *Consumer Reports*. July 2010. "Best Antidepressant for Anxiety According to Our Readers." *Consumer Reports*. Retrieved from: https://www.consumerreports.org/cro/2013/01/depression-and-anxiety/index.htm

P. 54
"The good news for women is that we're far more likely than men to seek professional . . ."
Donnelly, Laura. January 15, 2014. "Women Far More Likely than Men to Seek Counselling for Anxiety." *The Telegraph*. Retrieved from: https://www.telegraph.co.uk/news/10574941/Women-far-more-likely-than-men-to-seek-counselling-for-anxiety.html

P. 55
"Who's Who in Mental Health"
Mayo Clinic Staff. February 18, 2014. "Mental Health Providers: Tips on Finding One. Mayoclinic.org. Retrieved from: https://www.mayoclinic.org/diseases-conditions/mental-illness/in-depth/mental-health-providers/art-20045530

Beck's Anxiety Equation

P. 60
"So, here is Beck's equation . . ."
Saul, Helen. 2001. *Phobias: Fighting the Fear*. London: HarperCollins, page 264.

What I Think Is Making Me Anxious (Cognitive Behavioral Therapy)

P. 64
"According to Albert Ellis, creator of REBT (Rational Emotive Behavioral Therapy) . . ."
Ross, Will. 2006. "What Is Irrational?" REBT Network. Retrieved from: http://www.rebtnetwork.org/library/ideas.html

How I Think Is Making Me Anxious, Too (More Cognitive Behavioral Therapy)

P. 69
"The following ten 'cognitive distortions' or, in plain English, 'ten screwed up ways . . .'"
Burns, David D. 1999. *The Feeling Good Handbook*. New York: Plume.

A Reframe of Reframing: Byron Katie's "The Work"

P. 81
"In her own words, here's the story of how Byron Katie discovered 'The Work' . . ."
Editors of the Omega Institute. "4 Questions to Change Your Life: An Interview with Byron Katie, Creator of 'The Work.'" April 8, 2015. Huff-Post. Retrieved from: http://www.huffingtonpost.com/omega-institute-for-holistic-studies/4-questions-to-change-you_b_6926108.html

Ask Yourself Better Questions

P. 86
"As Tony Robbins says, 'Successful people …'"
Robbins, Tony. 1991. *Awaken the Giant Within: How to Take Control of Your Mental, Emotional, Physical and Financial Destiny.* New York: Summit Books, page 188.

P. 88
"Louise Hay recommends asking …"
Hay, Louise. November 25, 2011. "Say Yes." HealYourLife.com. Retrieved from: http://www.healyourlife.com/say-yes

The Importance of Not Being Perfekt

P. 90
"In her book *End the Struggle and Dance with Life*, Susan Jeffers …"
Jeffers, Susan. 1996. *End the Struggle and Dance with Life: How to Build Yourself Up When the World Gets You Down.* New York: St. Martin's Press, pages 36–42.

Let Go

P. 94
"The Five-Step Technique of the Sedona Method"
Dwoskin, Hale. 2007. *The Sedona Method: Your Key to Lasting Happiness, Success, Peace and Emotional Well-Being.* Sedona, Arizona: Sedona Press.

P. 96
"The first time I came across the idea of 'letting go' was in Shakti Gawain's …"
Gawain, Shakti. 1978. *Creative Visualization.* Berkeley: Whatever Publications, page 73.

Face Your Fears

P. 104
"I felt the same way, until I read a great book called . . ."
Jeffers, Susan. 1987. *Feel the Fear and Do It Anyway*. New York: Random House.

P. 105
"As Les Brown, the incredible motivational speaker . . .
www.Lesbrown.com

DIY Affirmations

P. 109
"I first ran across the idea of using affirmations in Louise Hay's book . . ."
Hay, Louise. 1984. *You Can Heal Your Life*. Santa Monica, California: Hay House.

Accentuate the Positive

P. 114
"According to an article in the *Atlantic*, "Men around us have continued to get . . ."
Kay, Katty, and Claire Shipman. May 2014. "The Confidence Gap." The *Atlantic*. Retrieved from: https://www.theatlantic.com/magazine/archive/2014/05/the-confidence-gap/359815/

P. 114
"And today women hold fewer than 19 percent of the board seats on Fortune . . ."
Peck, Emily. November 13, 2015. "Percentage of Women in Boardrooms Nears Milestone, but Has a Long Way to Go." HuffPost. Retrieved from: https://www.huffingtonpost.com/entry/women-corporate-boards_us_56450988e4b045bf3dee73cd

Just Do One Small Thing: The Art of Kaizen

P. 125
"In his book *One Small Step Can Change Your Life*, Robert Maurer, PhD ..."
Maurer, Robert, PhD. 2004. *One Small Step Can Change Your Life: The Kaizen Way*. New York: Workman Publishing Company.

Gratitude

P. 129
"How does gratitude work? Alex Korb, PhD, explains in his blog that our ..."
Korb, Alex, PhD. November 20, 2012. "The Grateful Brain." *Psychology Today*. Retrieved from: https://www.psychologytoday.com/us/blog/prefrontal-nudity/201211/the-grateful-brain

Faith

P. 134
"As you may or may not remember, Captain Scott O'Grady was an air force ..."
Claes, Bjorn. "One Amazing Kid—Capt. Scott O'Grady Escapes from Bosnia-Herzegovina." *F-16.Net*. Retrieved from: http://www.f-16.net/varia_article10.html

Just Breathe

P. 140
"This practice can be particularly helpful . . ."
Kinrys, Gustavo, and Lisa E. Wygant. October 2005. "Anxiety Disorders in Women: Does Gender Matter to Treatment?" *Revista Brasileira de Psiquiatria (Brazilian Journal of Psychiatry)*. Retrieved from: http://www.scielo.br/scielo.php?script=sci_arttext&pid=S1516-44462005000600003

P. 141
"This first method is called CO_2 rebreathing . . ."
Compiled by the Spire Wellness Team. September 19, 2017. "The Best Breathing Exercises for Anxiety." *Spire*. Retrieved from: https://medium.com/@spire.inc/the-best-breathing-exercises-for-anxiety -68cfdebfb461

P. 142
"I first read about the soft-belly technique in James S. Gordon's book . . ."
Gordon, James S., MD. 2008. *Unstuck*. New York: Penguin Press.

P. 143
"This breathing technique builds on the soft-belly . . ."
Brown, Richard P., MD, and Patricia Gerbarg, MD. 2012. *The Healing Power of the Breath: Simple Techniques to Reduce Stress and Anxiety, Enhance Concentration, and Balance Your Emotions*. Boston: Shambhala Publications.

P. 144
"Brown and Gerbarg's breath moving works exactly the way . . ."
Brown, Richard P., MD, and Patricia Gerbarg, MD. 2012. *The Healing Power of the Breath: Simple Techniques to Reduce Stress and Anxiety, Enhance Concentration, and Balance Your Emotions*. Boston: Shambhala Publications.

Meditate

P. 146
"A recent study done at Brown University found . . ."
Orenstein, David. April 20, 2017. "Mindfulness Class Helped Women, but Not Men, Overcome 'Negative Affect.'" Brown University. Retrieved from: https://news.brown.edu/articles/2017/04/meditation

P. 146
"Another study found menopausal women who used meditation reduced their hot flashes . . ."
Chang, Louise, MD, Reviewer. September 13, 2006. "Meditation May Cool Hot Flashes." WebMD. Retrieved from: https://www.webmd.com/menopause/news/20060913/meditation-may-cool-hot-flashes

P. 147
". . . meditation can be particularly helpful during pregnancy and birth."
Conner, Shannon. September 9, 2015. "Pregnancy Meditation: The Benefits of Mindfulness." Healthline. Retrieved from: https://www.healthline.com/health/pregnancy/meditation-benefits

P. 152
"Stephanie Vozza recommends some great ways to add mindful . . ."
Vozza, Stephanie. September 30, 2014. "Meditation Techniques for People Who Hate Meditation." *Fast Company*. Retrieved from: http://www.fastcompany.com/3036363/how-to-be-a-success-at-everything/meditation-techniques-for-people-who-hate-meditation

Sleep

P. 155
"According to an article on HuffPost . . ."
Huffington, Arianna, and Cindi Leive. December 6, 2017. "Sleep Challenge 2010: Women, It's Time to Sleep Our Way to the Top. Literally." *HuffPost*. Retrieved from: https://www.huffingtonpost.com/arianna-huffington/sleep-challenge-2010-wome_b_409973.html

P. 156
"Sixteen percent of us report missing one or more days a week . . ."
Boufis, Christina. March 11, 2011. "Why PMS Gives You Insomnia." WebMD. Retrieved from: https://www.webmd.com/women/pms/features/why-pms-gives-you-insomnia#1

P. 156
"Thirty-three percent of all women report insomnia . . ."
Boufis, Christina. March 11, 2011. "Why PMS Gives You Insomnia." WebMD. Retrieved from: https://www.webmd.com/women/pms/features/why-pms-gives-you-insomnia#1

P. 156
"...and 61 percent of us suffer sleep issues during both perimenopause and menopause."
Compiled by the National Sleep Foundation. Updated 2018. "Menopause and Sleep." National Sleep Foundation. Retrieved from: https://sleepfoundation.org/sleep-topics/menopause-and-sleep

P. 158
"But in her article 'Sleep Your Anxiety Away, Part I . . .'"
Hein, Becki A., MS, LPC. March 29, 2010. "Sleep Your Anxiety Away, Part I: You've Tried the Rest, Now Get Some Rest." GoodTherapy.org. Retrieved from: https://www.goodtherapy.org/blog/sleep-your-anxiety-away-part-I

P. 160
"Once you're comfortable, try Dr. Andrew Weil's simple . . ."
Weil, Andrew, MD. August 20, 2014. "The Simple Breathing Technique That Will Help You Sleep." *Prevention*. Retrieved from: https://www.prevention.com/health/sleep-energy/a20463313/breathing-exercise-for-insomnia/

Just Say No

P. 165
"What finally helped me tackle the challenge of learning to say no . . ."
Richardson, Cheryl. 1998. *Take Time for Your Life*. New York: Random House.

Slow Down

P. 170
"In her article 'How to Reduce Stress by Doing Less and Doing It Slowly' . . ."
Bernhard, Toni. "How to Reduce Stress by Doing Less and Doing It Slowly." *Tiny Buddha*. Retrieved from: http://tinybuddha.com/blog/how-to-reduce-stress-by-doing-less-and-doing-it-slowly

Laugh

P. 182
"According to Joseph Stromberg's article . . . in the *Smithsonian* . . ."
Stromberg, Joseph. July 31, 2012. "Simply Smiling Can Actually Reduce Stress." Smithsonianmag.com. Retrieved from: https://www.smithsonian mag.com/science-nature/simply-smiling-can-actually-reduce-stress -10461286/

P. 183
"Not only does laughter reduce the physical symptoms . . ."
Peterson, Tanya J. December 25, 2014. "Laughter Can Chase Away Anxiety." Healthy Place. Retrieved from: https://www.healthyplace.com/blogs/ anxiety-schmanxiety/2014/12/laughter-can-chase-away-anxiety/

P. 184
"Here are a couple of laughter yoga techniques taken from the book . . ."
McCloud, Ace. 2013. *Laughter and Humor Therapy*. San Bernardino, California: self-published.

Play

P. 187
"According to Lawrence Robinson's article on HelpGuide.org . . ."
Robinson, Lawrence, Melinda Smith, MA, Jeanne Segal, PhD, and Jennifer Shubin. Updated June 2019. "The Benefits of Play for Adults." HelpGuide. org. Retrieved from: http://www.helpguide.org/articles/emotional-health/ benefits-of-play-for-adults.htm

Music

P. 192
"As Jane Collingwood writes in her article for Psych Central . . ."
Collingwood, Jane. Updated October 8, 2018. "The Power of Music to Reduce Stress." Psych Central. Retrieved from: http://psychcentral.com/ lib/the-power-of-music-to-reduce-stress/

P. 192

"And now we have some research that tells us that listening to music affects men and women differently. . ."
Sax, Leonard. 2005. *Why Gender Matters: What Parents and Teachers Need to Know About the Emerging Science of Sex Differences.* New York: Doubleday, page 16.

P. 193

"According to Susan Kuchinskas, writing for WebMD . . ."
Kuchinskas, Susan. October 7, 2010. "How Making Music Reduces Stress." WebMD. Retrieved from: https://www.webmd.com/balance/stress-management/features/how-making-music-reduces-stress#1

Love Your Body

P. 195

"A study done by *Glamour* on how women . . ."
Dreisbach, Shaun. February 3, 2011. "Shocking Body-Image News: 97% of Women Will Be Cruel to Their Bodies Today." *Glamour.* Retrieved from: https://www.glamour.com/story/shocking-body-image-news-97-percent-of-women-will-be-cruel-to-their-bodies-today

P. 195

"Over the course of our lifetimes, women . . ."
Kratofil, Colleen. March 30, 2017. "Can You Guess How Much a Woman Spends on Her Makeup in Her Lifetime? (We Were Way Off!)" *People.* Retrieved from: https://www. people.com/style/how-much-does-a-woman -spend-on-makeup/

P. 195

"And a *TODAY/AOL* body-image survey found . . .
Dahl, Melissa. February 24, 2014. "Stop Obsessing: Women Spend 2 Weeks a Year on Their Appearance, *TODAY* Survey Shows." *TODAY.* Retrieved from: https://www.today.com/health/stop-obsessing-women-spend-2-weeks-year-their-appearance-today-2D12104866

P. 195
"While there's no doubt that men judge women on their appearance . . ."
Barber, Nigel, PhD. May 2, 2013. "Why Women Feel Bad About Their Appearance." *Psychology Today.* Retrieved from: https://www.psychologytoday.com/us/blog/the-human-beast/201305/why-women-feel -bad-about-their-appearance

P. 196
"We use that fear of not looking 'good enough' . . ."
Barber, Nigel, PhD. May 2, 2013. "Why Women Feel Bad About Their Appearance." *Psychology Today.* Retrieved from: https://www.psychologytoday.com/us/blog/the-human-beast/201305/why-women-feel-bad -about-their-appearance

P. 196
"The therapist also helped them see that . . ."
Dreisbach, Shaun. February 3, 2011. "Shocking Body-Image News: 97% of Women Will Be Cruel to Their Bodies Today." *Glamour.* Retrieved from: https://www.glamour.com/story/shocking-body-image-news-97-percent-of-women-will-be-cruel-to-their-bodies-today

Get Moving

P. 200
"An article from the Anxiety and Depression Association . . ."
"Exercise for Stress and Anxiety." Anxiety and Depression Association of America. Retrieved from: https://adaa.org/living-with-anxiety/ managing-anxiety/exercise-stress-and-anxiety

P. 201
"So why are 60 percent of women in this country not getting the recommended two and a half hours . . ."

Lambert, Tarla. August 27, 2017. "Study Finds High Rates of Anxiety in Women." Women's Agenda. Retrieved from: https://womensagenda.com.au/leadership/advice/new-study-links-anxiety-levels-lack-exercise-among-young-busy-women/

Keep Moving, Stay Motivated

P. 209
"Research shows women are far more likely than men to say they lack the willpower . . ."
Compiled by the APA. 2010. "Gender and Stress." American Psychological Association. Retrieved from: http://www.apa.org/news/press/releases/stress/2010/gender-stress.aspx

P. 210
"In his book *The Power of Habit*, Charles Duhigg explores the . . ."
Duhigg, Charles. 2012. *The Power of Habit: Why We Do What We Do in Life and Business*. New York: Random House.

Yoga

P. 215
". . . yoga has been scientifically proven to significantly reduce anxiety . . ."
Javnbakht, M., R. Hejazi Kenari, and M. Ghasemi. March 20, 2009. "Effects of Yoga on Depression and Anxiety of Women." *Complimentary Therapies in Clinical Practice*. Retrieved from: https://www.ncbi.nlm.nih.gov/pubmed/19341989

P. 215
"Yoga has also been proven to be useful in calming . . ."
Attre, Shalini. Oct. 27, 2015. "Get Guaranteed Relief from Painful PMS with Yoga!" Nirogam.com. Retrieved from: http://hindi.nirogam.com/yoga-relief-pre-menstrual-sydrome/

P. 216
"I've taken most of the following postures (asanas) from the book *Yoga as Medicine . . .*"
McCall, Timothy, MD. 2007. *Yoga as Medicine.* New York: Bantam Dell.

P. 219
"It can also be safely done in pregnancy."
Felder, Lynn. August 28, 2007. "Prenatal Yoga Poses for Each Trimester." *Yoga Journal.* Retrieved from: https://www.yogajournal.com/practice/yoga-for-moms-to-be

Qigong

P. 225
"And research shows that qigong is particularly useful . . ."
Compiled by Omega Institute for Holistic Studies. February 19, 2015. "Managing Menopause with Qigong." Omega. Retrieved from: https://www.eomega.org/article/managing-menopause-with-qigong

P. 225
"The following exercises are my favorites from the excellent book *The Qigong Workbook . . .*"
Lam, Kam Chuen. 2014. *The Qigong Workbook for Anxiety.* Oakland: New Harbinger Publications, Inc.

Acupressure

P. 233
"The following techniques come from the book . . ."
Gach, Michael Reed, PhD, and Beth Ann Henning. 2004. *Acupressure for Emotional Healing.* New York: Bantam Dell.

P. 242
"This technique can be used to calm anxiety . . ."
Cassileth, Barrie, PhD. July 30, 2018. "Complimentary Therapies in Cancer Care: Acupressure." *Cancer Connect.* Retrieved from: https://news.

cancerconnect.com/treatment-care/complimentary-therapies-in-cancer-care-acupressure-Zooc-yXnsUuEwAxNHcZ-Ag

EFT: Emotional Freedom Technique, or Tapping

P. 244
"According to Gary Craig, the man who developed EFT . . ."
Craig, Gary. "Gold Standard of EFT Tapping Therapy." Retrieved from: http://www.emofree.com

P. 244
"In a study published in the *Journal of Nervous and Mental Disease* . . ."
Church, Dawson, PhD, Garret Yount, PhD, and Audrey Brooks, PhD. October 2012. "The Effect of Emotional Freedom Techniques on Stress Biochemistry: A Randomized Controlled Trial." *Journal of Nervous and Mental Disease* vol. 200, no. 10, pages 891–896. Retrieved from: https://www.ncbi.nlm.nih.gov/pubmed/22986277

Heal with Water

P. 251
"According to Amanda Carlson, RD, 'Studies have shown that . . .'
Shaw, Gina. July 7, 2009. "Water and Stress Reduction: Sipping Stress Away." WebMD. Retrieved from: http://www.webmd.com/diet/water -stress-reduction

P. 252
"If so, here are some great suggestions from Monica Nelson's . . ."
Nelson, Monica. September 13, 2013. "How to Drink More Water Each Day." *U.S. News & World Report*. Retrieved from: https://health .usnews.com/health-news/blogs/eat-run/2013/09/13/how-to-drink -more-water-each-day

P. 253

"Research appearing in the *Journal of Complementary Therapies in Medicine*
..."
Editors of *Prevention*. September 14, 2015. "5 Reasons You Need to Take a Bath
Tonight (No Matter How Busy You Are)." Prevention.com. Retrieved from:
http://www.prevention.com/mind-body/natural-remedies/science
-backed-reasons-take-bath

P. 253

"... they can enjoy the comfort of a warm bath ..."
Compiled by University of Arkansas for Medical Science. March 8, 2019.
"Can Pregnant Women Take Baths?" UAMS Health. Retrieved from:
https://uamshealth.com/healthlibrary2/medicalmyths/pregnantwomen
takebaths/

P. 254

"If you're interested in reading more about the comfort of bathing ..."
Louden, Jennifer. 1992. *The Woman's Comfort Book*. New York: Harper
Collins.

P. 254

"As it says in the article 'How Does Nature Impact Our Wellbeing?' ..."
Larson, Jean, PhD, CTRS, HTR, and Mary Jo Kreitzer, RN, PhD.
(Reviewers) June 25, 2014. "How Does Nature Impact Our Wellbeing?"
University of Minnesota. Retrieved from: https://www.takingcharge.csh.
umn.edu/how-does-nature-impact-our-wellbeing

Nourish Yourself

P. 255

"Studies show that women are much more likely than men to ..."
Compiled by the American Psychological Association. 2010. "Gender and
Stress." *American Psychological Association*. Retrieved from: http://www.apa.
org/news/press/releases/stress/2010/gender-stress.aspx

Eat and Drink This

P. 260
"As Caroline Cassels writes in her article 'Whole Diet May Ward Off . . .'"
Cassels, Caroline. January 15, 2010. "Whole Diet May Ward Off Depression and Anxiety." Medscape.com. Retrieved from: https://www.medscape.com/viewarticle/715239

P. 260
"Daniel K. Hall-Flavin, MD, recommends the following rules for . . ."
Hall-Flavin, Daniel, MD. March 6, 2014. "Is It True That Certain Foods Worsen Anxiety and Others Have a Calming Effect?" MayoClinic. Retrieved from: http://www.mayoclinic.org/diseases-conditions/generalized-anxiety-disorders/expert/answers-coping-with-anxiety/faq-20057987

P. 261
"In her article '9 Foods That Help or Hurt Anxiety' in *Everyday Health*, Beth W. Orenstein recommends . . ."
Orenstein, Beth, W. April 7, 2014. "9 Foods That Help or Hurt Anxiety." Everydayhealth.com. Retrieved from: https://www.everydayhealth.com/anxiety-pictures/anxiety-foods-that-help-foods-that-hurt-0118.aspx

P. 263
"If you're looking for a little something extra you can do to help . . ."
Oz, Mehmet MD. March 12, 2012. "Dr. Oz's Worry Cure and Diet Plan." Doctoroz.com. Retrieved from: https://www.doctoroz.com/article/dr-ozs-worry-cure-diet-plan

P. 263
"As Dr. William Cole writes. . ."
Cole, William, DC. September 25, 2014. "13 Foods to Help Ease Anxiety & Stress." Mindbodygreen.com. Retrieved from: http://www.mindbodygreen.com/0-15428/13-foods-to-help-ease-anxiety-stress.html

Don't Eat or Drink This

P. 264
"As Shelly Guillory writes in her article for Livestrong . . .
Guillory, Shelly. January 28, 2015. "Foods That Trigger Anxiety." Livestrong.
com.

P. 265
"Caffeine Intoxication Diagnostic Criteria"
American Psychiatric Association. 2013. *Diagnostic and Statistical Manual of Mental Disorders: DSM-5*. Washington, DC: American Psychiatric Association, page 506.

P. 266
"Here are some of the most common sources of caffeine . . ."
Edited by the staff of IFIC Review. May 1, 2008. "Caffeine and Health: Clarifying the Controversies." International Food Information Council Foundation. Retrieved from: https://www.foodinsight.org/wp-content/uploads/2008/05/Caffeine_v8-2.pdf

Journal

P. 272
"According to Barbara Markway, PhD, 'One of the most useful things . . .'"
Markway, Barbara, PhD. April 13, 2014. "How to Keep a Thought Diary to Combat Anxiety." *Psychology Today*. Retrieved from: https://www.psychologytoday.com/us/blog/shyness-is-nice/201404/how-keep-thought-diary-combat-anxiety

Plan to Worry

P. 276
"According to Joe Brownstein's article . . ."
Brownstein, Joe. July 26, 2011. "Planning, Worry, Time May Help Ease Anxiety." *Live Science*. Retrieved from: https://www.livescience.com/15233-planning-worry-time-ease-anxiety.html

Get Organized

P. 281
"In a survey done on behalf of HuffPost . . ."
Compiled by HuffPost. May 22, 2013. "Home Organization Is Major Source of Stress for Americans, Survey Finds." *HuffPost*. Retrieved from: https://www.huffingtonpost.com/2013/05/22/home-organization-stress -survey_n_3308575.html

Do Good, Feel Better

P. 292
"According to Mary Ann Christie Burnside's article . . ."
Burnside, Mary Ann Christie. March 22, 2011. "Intentional Acts of Kindness." *Mindful*. Retrieved from: http://www.mindful.org/intentional -acts-of-kindness/

Acknowledgments

THERE ARE so many people who helped make this book possible.

First and foremost, I would like to thank my mother, Shirley M. Buck. She was one of the first people to read this book, and although she didn't live to see the book published, she was one of my biggest cheerleaders along the way.

I would also like to thank Tyler Leeds, Lisa Leeds, Grant Leeds, Molly Leeds, and Marilyn Gfroerer, who were always there for me.

I would like to thank my amazing coaches, Peg Doyle, Suzan Czajkowski, and Andrea Novakowski. Thank you all for all your help and support along the way. You're the best.

I feel very lucky to have a great team to have supported, suggested, and helped me along the way: Gail Morokowski and Sharon Tousley. And a big thanks to Meg Joyce for the beautiful illustrations. Thanks also to Chad Beckerman for the beautiful cover.

Thanks to my wonderful editor, Lindsey Alexander, who helped make this book a reality. Thanks also to Salvatore Borriello, Penina Lopez, and Andrea Reider, who helped make the book better.

I would like to thank my talented, patient writers' group, who read and suggested and guided me along the way: Patricia Barletta, Linda Grochowalski, Wendy Rogalinski, DeAnna Putnam, and Marcia Withiam Wilson.

Thanks also to my wonderful friends for their support, for their great suggestions, and for being such an important part of this process: Susan Conti, Sharon Winn, Roberta Rosenthal Hawkins, Marcia Martin, and Linda DeRensis. And to my gifted professional colleagues, Hollis Burkhart, Michelle Harris, and Sister Jacqueline LeBoeuf. I feel lucky to know you all.

About the Author

WENDY LEEDS is anxious.

As a three-time cancer survivor, she is an expert on what it's like to live with anxiety.

As an experienced, licensed psychotherapist, Wendy's mission is to help anxious women learn to acknowledge and ease their anxieties. Her work empowers women to create the calm, centered lives they were born to live.

Wendy lives in Massachusetts with her husband, Tom, and their dog, Myles Standish.

To learn more about her work and to connect with her directly, visit www.WendyLeeds.com.